INTRODUCTION

It was the following letter from Mr. William Louden to the editor of ~"Health Culture"~ which prompted the author to issue the ~"Nature Cure Magazine"~ (published from November, 1907, to October, 1909). In the series of books of which this is the first volume, he will endeavor to collect and systematize all his former writings in the~ "Nature Cure Magazine," "Health Culture," "Life and Action,"~ the ~"Naturopath,"~ the ~"Volksrath,"~ and other publications, and to amplify these by new material obtained through further research and wider experience.

Mr. Albert Turner,

Editor of ~"Health Culture."~

DEAR SIR—I write to ask what you consider the best book or pamphlet to put into the hands of people generally, in regard to the preservation of health. I know ther e are a number of very excellent publications, but as a rule they deal with certain details or phases of the question, and do not begin with the great underlying principles in such a way as to attract and hold the attention of the masses. One advocates one plan, and another an entirely different, and sometimes a directly opposite plan—such as uncooked vs. thoroughly cooked food; a strictly vegetarian diet, and mental culture in place of attention to either, etc. Such a state of affairs makes it confusing to average people and gets them to believe that health reformers are all at sea, and what is good for one is not good for another, or, in common language, "what is one man's meat is another's poison."

Now, I know it is natural, and doubtless best, that there should be a difference of opinion on any question, but at the same time, if any movement is to be crowned with great success, there should be some underlying principles upon which all should agree, and these should be pressed to the forefront, so as to attract and hold the attention of the people, in place of the divergent details upon which they disagree. If these fundamental laws and principles are thoroughly studied and well defined, it may be found that they would explain the discrepancies between the different theories, and that under certain conditions, one plan is best, and that under different conditions another plan is more applicable, etc. The pushing of these fundamental principles to the front would also tend to correct errors into which the different theorists have fallen, and would certainly tend to make the different theories more homogeneous and more easily understood by people in general, than at present.

In my opinion, the general fundamental principles of life and health are what people need to understand more than anything else. Without this, most of the details will be meaningless or at least confusing dogmas. I don't mean by these fundamental principles the details of anatomy, or, for that matter, the details of anything else, but the general rules governing life and death, so that people may know which way they, are tending, and may understand the many illusions with which life and death, as well as all else in nature are beset.

The present volume and others of the "Nature Cure Series" which are to follow are an attempt to answer Mr. Louden's inquiry and to formulate and elucidate the fundamental laws of health, disease and cure for which he and many others have been vainly seeking. Who among you at some time or another, has not thought and felt like Mr. Louden and in doubt and perplexity voiced Pilate's query,

What Is Truth?

The exact information and rational method of teaching which Mr. Louden is seeking, has heretofore been wanting in health-culture literature.

Many, indeed, stand ready and willing to show the way to physical, mental and moral perfection. Hundreds, yes, thousands, of different cults, isms, teachers, books and periodicals treat of these subjects, but their teachings are so manifold, so contradictory and confusing, that one becomes bewildered amid the ever increasing testimony. As is often the case in the study of complicated subjects, the more one reads and the more one hears, the less one knows. I believe that no one has described more strikingly this state of general perplexity than Mr. Louden in his excellent letter.

Nevertheless, these simple fundamental laws and principles really exist. They must exist, because everything in Nature, including the processes of health, of disease and cure, of birth, of life and death, are subject to law and order.

Allopathy, or Old School Medical Science, admits that it does not know these fundamental principles; that it reasons, not from underlying causes, but from external symptoms and personal experiences. It is, therefore, self-confessedly full of doubts, errors and confusion; in short, empirical—and necessarily, a failure.

Many teachers of Nature Cure, Hygiene and Health cults have stumbled accidentally upon some of the natural laws and true methods of healing, but have failed to grasp and to formulate the broad underlying principles. For this reason they are often partly right and partly wrong and very apt to overdo certain methods to the neglect of others just as effective and essential, or even more so.

I shall endeavor in these volumes to formulate and elucidate some of the fundamental laws and principles underlying the phenomena of life and death, health, disease and cure, and shall try to ascertain in the light of these laws how much of truth and how much of error, how much of usefulness and how much of harmfulness there may be contained in the various theories and systems of living and of healing.

Nature Owe an Exact Science

One of the reasons why Nature Cure is not more popular with the medical profession and the public is that it is too simple. The average mind is more impressed by the involved and mysterious than by the simple and common-sense.

However, it remains a fact that "exact science" reduces complexity and confusion to simplicity and clearness. Science becomes exact science only when the underlying laws which correlate and unify its scattered facts and theories have been discovered.

These simple laws rightly understood and applied will do for medical science what the law of gravitation has done for physics and astronomy, and what the laws of chemical affinity have done for chemistry, they will place medical science in the ranks of exact sciences. The understanding and proper application of these truths will explain every fact and phenomenon in the processes of health, disease and cure, and will enable the student to reason from simple, natural laws and principles to their logical effects. The "Regular" school of medicine, so far, has endeavored to build a medical science on the observation of "effects" and "experiences," but since one fundamental law of nature may produce a million seemingly differing effects it becomes self-evident that it is utterly impossible to found an exact science on such uncertain and conflicting evidence.

The primary laws and principles once understood, it becomes easy to reason from and to explain through them, the various phenomena which they produce. Herein lie the merit and achievement of the Nature Cure philosophy.

Chapter I

What ~Is~ Nature Cure?

It is vastly more than a system of curing aches and pains; it is a complete revolution in the art and science of living. It is the practical realization and application of all that is good in natural science, philosophy and religion. Like many another world-wide revolution and reformation, it had its inception in Germany, the land of thinkers and philosophers.

About seventy years ago this greatest and most beneficent of reformation movements was inaugurated by Priessnitz in Grafenberg, a small village in the Silesian mountains. The originator of Nature Cure was a simple farmer, but he had a natural genius for the art of healing.

His pharmacopeia consisted not in poisonous pills and potions but in plenty of exercise, fresh mountain air, water treatments in the cool, sparkling brooks, and simple, wholesome country fare, consisting largely of black bread, vegetables, and milk fresh from cows fed on nutritious mountain grasses.

The results accomplished by these simple means were wonderful. Before he died, a large sanitarium, filled with patients from all over the world and from all stations of life, had grown up around his forest home.

Among those who made the pilgrimage to Grafenberg to become patients and students of this genial healer, the simple-minded farmer-physician, were wealthy merchants, princes and doctors from all parts of the world.

Rapidly the idea of drugless healing spread over Germany and over the civilized world. In the Fatherland, Hahn the apothecary, Kuhne the weaver, Rikli the manufacturer, Father Kneipp the priest, Lahmann the doctor, and Turnvater Jahn, the founder of physical culture, became enthusiastic pupils and followers of Priessnitz.

Each one of these men enlarged and enriched some special field of the great realm of natural healing. Some elaborated the water cure and natural dietetics, others invented various systems of manipulative treatment, earth, air and light cures, magnetic healing, mental therapeutics, curative gymnastics, etc., etc. Von Peckzely added the Diagnosis from the Eye, which reveals not only the innermost secrets of the human organism, but also Nature's ways and means of cure, and the changes for better or for worse continually occurring in the body.

In this country, Dr. Trall of New York, Dr. Jackson of Danville, Dr. Kellogg of Battle Creek, and others caught the infection and crossed the ocean to become students of Priessnitz. The achievements of these men in their respective fields of endeavor will stand as enduring monuments to the eternal truths revealed by the genius of Nature Cure.

Quimby, the itinerant spiritualist and healer, became successful and renowned by the application of the natural methods of cure. At first his favorite methods were water, massage, magnetic and mental treatment. Gradually he concentrated his efforts on metaphysical methods of cure, and before he died, he evolved a complete system of magnetic and mental therapeutics.

Quimby's teachings and methods were adopted by Mrs. Eddy, his most enthusiastic pupil, and by her elaborated into Christian Science, the latest and most successful of modern mental-healing cults.

Dr. Still of Kirksville, Missouri, made a valuable addition to natural methods of treatment by the invention of Osteopathy, a system of scientific manipulation of the bony structures, nerves and nerve centers, muscles and ligaments. A later development of manipulative science is Chiropractic, originated by Dr. Palmer of Davenport, Iowa. Thus the simple pioneers of German Nature Cure, every one of them gifted by Nature with the instinct and genius of the true healer, who is born, not made, laid the foundation for the worldwide modern healthculture movement.

They were not blinded or confused by the conflicting theories of books and authorities, or by the action of a thousand different drugs on a legion of different symptoms, but applied common-sense reasoning to the solution of the problems of health, disease and cure.

They went for inspiration to field and forest rather than to the murky atmosphere of the dissecting and vivisection rooms. They studied the whole and not only the parts, causes as well as effects and symptoms. Realizing that man had lost his natural instinct and strayed far from Nature's ways, they studied and imitated the natural habits of the animal creation rather than the confusing doctrines of the schools.

Thus they proclaimed the "return to Nature" and the "new gospel of health," which are destined to free humanity from the destructive influences of alcoholism, red meat overeating, the dope and tobacco habit, and of drug poisoning, vaccination, surgical mutilation, vivisection and a thousand other abuses practiced in the name of science.

When parents learn how to create children in accord with natural law, how to mold their bodies and their characters into harmony and beauty before the new life sees the light of day, when they learn to rear their offspring in health of body and purity of mind in harmony with the laws of their being, then we shall have true types of beautiful manhood and womanhood, then children will no longer be a curse and a burden to themselves and to those who bring them into the world or to society at large.

These thoughts are not the mere dreams of a visionary. When we see the wonderful changes wrought in a human being by a few months or years of rational living and treatment, it seems not impossible or improbable that these ideals may be realized within a few generations.

Children thus born and reared in harmony with the law will be the future masters of the earth. They will need neither gold nor influence to win in the race of life—their innate powers of body and soul will make them victors over every circumstance. The offspring of alcoholism, drug poisoning and sexual perversity will cut but sorry figures in comparison with the manhood and womanhood of a true and noble aristocracy of health.

Chapter II

Catechism of Nature Cure

The philosophy of Nature Cure is based on sciences dealing with newly discovered or rediscovered natural laws and principles, and with their application to the phenomena of life and death, health, disease and cure.

Every new science embodying new modes of thought requires exact modes of expression and new definitions of already well-known words and phrases.

Therefore, we have endeavored to define, as precisely as possible, certain words and phrases which convey meanings and ideas peculiar to the teachings of Nature Cure.

The student of Nature Cure and kindred subjects will do well to study these definitions and formulated principles closely, as they contain the pith and marrow of our philosophy and greatly facilitate its understanding.

(1) What Is Nature Cure?

Nature Cure is a system of building the entire being in harmony with the constructive principle in Nature on the physical, mental, moral and spiritual planes of being.

(2) What Is the Constructive Principle in Nature?

The constructive principle in Nature is that principle which builds up, improves and repairs, which always makes for the perfect type, whose activity in Nature is designated as evolutionary and constructive and which is opposed to the destructive principle in Nature

(3) What Is the Destructive Principle in Nature?

The destructive principle in Nature is that principle which disintegrates and destroys existing forms and types, and whose activity in Nature is designated as devolutionary and destructive.

(4) What Is Normal or Natural?

That is normal or natural which is in harmonic relation with the life purposes of the individual and the constructive principle in Nature.

(5) What Is Health?

Health is normal and harmonious vibration of the elements and forces composing the human entity on the physical, mental, moral and spiritual planes of being, in conformity with the constructive principle of Nature applied to individual life.

(6) What Is Disease?

Disease is abnormal or inharmonious vibration of the elements and forces composing the human entity on one or more planes of being, in conformity with the destructive principle of Nature applied to individual life.

(7) What Is the Primary Cause of Disease?

The primary cause of disease, barring accidental or surgical injury to the human organism and surroundings hostile to human life, is violation of Nature's Laws.

(8) What Is the Effect of Violation of Nature's Laws on the Physical Human Organism?

The effect of violation of Nature's Laws on the physical human organism are:

Lowered vitality. Abnormal composition of blood and lymph. Accumulation of waste matter, morbid materials and poisons.

These conditions are identical with disease, because they tend to lower, hinder or inhibit normal function (harmonious vibration) and because they engender and promote destruction of living tissues.

(9) What Is Acute Disease?

What is commonly called acute disease is in reality the result of Nature's efforts to eliminate from the organism waste matter, foreign matter and poisons, and to repair injury to living tissues. In other words, every so-called acute disease is the result of a cleansing and healing effort of Nature. The real disease is lowered vitality, abnormal composition of the vital fluids (blood and lymph) and the resulting accumulation of waste materials and poisons.

(10) What Is Chronic Disease?

Chronic disease is a condition of the organism in which lowered vibration (lowered vitality), due to the accumulation of waste matter and poisons, with the consequent destruction of vital parts and organs, has progressed to such an extent that Nature's constructive and healing forces are no longer able to react against the disease conditions by acute corrective efforts (healing crises). Chronic disease is a condition of the organismin which the morbid encumbrances have gained the ascendancy and prevent acute reaction (healing crises) on the part of the constructive forces of Nature. Chronic disease is the inability of the organism to react by acute efforts or healing crises against constitutional disease conditions.

(11) What Is a Healing Crisis?

A healing crisis is an acute reaction, resulting from the ascendancy of Nature's healing forces over disease conditions. Its tendency is toward recovery, and it is, therefore, in conformity with Nature's constructive principle.

(12) Are All Acute Reactions Healing Crises?

No, there are healing crises and disease crises.

(13) What Is a Disease Crisis?

A disease crisis is an acute reaction resulting from the ascendancy of disease conditions over the healing forces of the organism. Its tendency is toward fatal termination, and it is, therefore, in conformity with Nature's destructive principle

(14) What Is Cure?

Cure is the readjustment of the human organism from abnormal to normal conditions and functions.

(15) What Methods of Cure Are in Conformity with the Constructive Principle in Nature?

Those methods which:

Establish normal surroundings and natural habits of life in accord with Nature's Laws. Economize vital force. Build up the blood on a natural basis, that is, supply the blood with its natural constituents in right proportions. Promote the elimination of waste matter and poisons without in any way injuring the human body. Arouse the individual in the highest possible degree to the consciousness of personal accountability and the necessity of intelligent personal effort and self-help.

(16) Are Medicines in Conformity with the Constructive Principle in Nature?

Medicines are in conformity with the constructive principle in Nature insofar as they, in themselves, are not injurious and destructive to the human organism and insofar as they act as tissue foods and promote the neutralization and elimination of morbid matter and poisons.

(17) Are Poisonous Drugs and Promiscuous Surgical Operations in Conformity with the Constructive Principle in Nature?

Poisonous drugs and promiscuous operations are not usually in conformity with the constructive principle in Nature, because:

They suppress acute diseases or reactions (crises), the cleaning and healing efforts of Nature. They are in themselves harmful and destructive to human life. Such treatment fosters the belief that drugs and surgical operations can be substituted for obedience to Nature's Laws and for personal effort and self-help.

(18) Is Metaphysical Healing in Conformity with the Constructive Principle in Nature?

Metaphysical systems of healing are in conformity with the constructive principle in Nature insofar as:

They do not interfere with or suppress Nature's healing efforts. They awaken hope and confidence (therapeutic faith) and increase the inflow of vital force into the organism.

They are not in conformity with the constructive principle in Nature in so far as:

They fail to assist Nature's healing efforts. They ignore, obscure and deny the laws of Nature and defy the dictates of reason and common sense. They substitute, in the treatment of disease, a blind, dogmatic belief in the wonder-working power of metaphysical formulas and prayer for intelligent cooperation with Nature's constructive forces for personal effort and self-help. They weaken the consciousness of personal responsibility.

(19) Is Nature Cure in Conformity with the Constructive Principle in Nature?

Nature Cure is in conformity with the constructive principle in Nature because:

It teaches that the primary cause of weakness and disease is disobedience to the laws of Nature. It arouses the individual to the study of natural laws and demonstrates the necessity of strict compliance with these laws. It strengthens the consciousness of personal responsibility of the individual for his own status of health and for the hereditary conditions, traits and tendencies of his off-spring. It encourages personal effort and self-help. It adapts surroundings and habits of life to natural laws. It assists Nature's cleansing and healing efforts by simple natural means and methods of treatment which are in no wise harmful or destructive to health and life, and which are within the reach of everyone.

(20) What Are the Natural Methods of Living and of Treatment?

Return to Nature by the regulation of eating, drinking, breathing, bathing, dressing, working, resting, thinking, the moral life, sexual and social activities, etc., on a normal and natural basis. Elementary remedies, such as water, air, light, earth cures, magnetism, electricity, etc. Chemical remedies, such as scientific food selection and combination, specific nutritional augmentation with natural food concentrates, homeopathic medicines, simple herb extracts and the vitochemical remedies. Mechanical remedies, such as corrective gymnastics, massage, magnetic treatment, chiropractic or osteopathic manipulation and, when indicated, surgery. Mental and spiritual remedies, such as scientific relaxation, normal suggestion, constructive thought, the prayer of faith, etc.

Chapter III

What Is Life?

In our study of the cause and character of disease we must endeavor to begin at the beginning, and that is with LIFE itself, for the processes of health, disease and cure are manifestations of that which we call life, vitality, life elements, etc.

While endeavoring to fathom the mystery of life we soon realize, however, that we are dealing with an ultimate which no human mind is capable of solving or explaining. We can study and understand life only in its manifestations, not in its origin and real essence.

There are two prevalent, but widely differing, conceptions of the nature of life or vital force: the material and the vital.

The former looks upon life or vital force with all its physical, mental and psychical phenomena as manifestations of the electric, magnetic and chemical activities of the physical-material elements composing the human organism. From this viewpoint, life is a sort of spontaneous combustion, or, as one scientist expressed it, a succession of fermentations.

This materialistic conception of life, however, has already become obsolete among the more advanced biologists as a result of the wonderful discoveries of modern science, which are fast bridging the chasm between the material and the spiritual realms of being.

But medical science, as taught in the regular schools, is still dominated by the old, crude, mechanical conception of vital force and this, as we shall see, accounts for some of its gravest errors of theory and of practice.

The vital conception of life, on the other hand, regards it as the primary force of all forces, coming from the great central source of all power.

This force, which permeates, heats and animates the entire created universe, is the expression of the divine will, the "logos," the "word" of the great creative intelligence. It is this divine energy which sets in motion the whirls in the ether, the electric corpuscles and ions that make up the different atoms and elements of matter.

These corpuscles and ions are positive and negative forms of electricity. Electricity is a form of energy. It is intelligent energy; otherwise it could not move with that same wonderful precision in the electrons of the atoms as in the suns and planets of the sidereal universe.

This intelligent energy can have but one source: the will and the intelligence of the Creator; as Swedenborg expresses it, "the great central sun of the universe."

If this supreme intelligence should withdraw its energy, the electrical charges (forms of energy) and with it the atoms, elements, and the entire material universe would disappear in the flash of a moment.

From this it appears that crude matter, instead of being the source of life and of all its complicated mental and spiritual phenomena (which assumption, on the face of it, is absurd), is only an expression of the Life Force, itself a manifestation of the great creative intelligence which some call God, others Nature, the Oversoul, Brahma, Prana, etc., each one according to his best understanding.

It is this supreme power and intelligence, acting in and through every atom, molecule and cell in the human body, which is the true healer, the vis medicatrix nature, which always endeavors to repair, to heal and to restore the perfect type. All that the physician can do is to remove obstructions and to establish normal conditions within and around the patient, so that the healer within can do his work to the best advantage.

Here the Christian Scientist will say: "That is exactly what we claim. All is God, all is mind! There is no matter! Our attitude toward disease is based on these facts."

Well, what of it, Brother Scientist? Suppose, in the final analysis, matter is nothing but vibration, an expression of Divine Mind and Will. That, for all practical purposes, does not justify me to deny and to ignore its reality.

Because I have an "all-mind" body, is it advisable for me to place myself in the way of an "all-mind" locomotive moving at the rate of sixty miles an hour?

The question is not what matter is in the final analysis, but how matter affects us. We have to take it and treat it as we find it. We must be as obedient to the laws of matter as to those of the higher planes of being.

Life Is Vibratory

In the final analysis, all things in Nature, from a fleeti g thought or emotion to the hardest piece of diamond or platinum, are modes of motion or vibration. A few years ago physical science assumed that an atom was the smallest imaginable part of a given element of matter; that although infinitesimally small, it still represented solid matter. Now, in the light of better evidence, we have good reason to believe that there is no such thing as solid matter: that every atom is made up of charges of negative and positive electricity acting in and upon an omnipresent ether; that the difference between an atom of iron and of hydrogen or any other element consists solely in the number of electrical charges or corpuscles it contains, and on the velocity with which these vibrate around one another.

Thus the atom, which was thought to be the ultimate particle of solid matter, is found to be a little universe in itself in which corpuscles of electricity rotate or vibrate around one another like the suns and planets in the sidereal universe. This explains what we mean when we say life and matter are vibratory.

As early as 1863 John Newlands discovered that when he arranged the elements of matter in the order of their atomic weight, they displayed the same relationship to one another as do the tones in the musical scale. Thus modern chemistry demonstrates the verity of the music of the spheres—

another visionary concept of ancient mysticism. The individual atoms in themselves, as well as all the atoms of matter in their relationship to one another, are constructed and arranged in exact correspondence with the laws of harmony. Therefore the entire sidereal universe is built on the laws of music.

That which is orderly, lawful, good, beautiful, natural, healthy, vibrates in unison with the harmonics of this great "Diapason of Nature"; in other words, it is in alignment with the constructive principle in Nature.

That which is disorderly, abnormal, ugly, unnatural, unhealthy, vibrates in discord with Nature's harmonics. It is in alignment with the destructive principle in Nature.

What we call "Inanimate Nature" is beautiful and orderly because it plays in tune with the score of the Symphony of Life. Man alone can play out of tune. This is his privilege, if he so chooses, by virtue of his freedom of choice and action.

We can now better understand the definitions of health and of disease, given in Chapter Two, "Catechism of Nature Cure" as follows:

"Health is normal and harmonious vibration of the elements and forces composing the human entity on the physical, mental, moral and spiritual planes of being, in conformity with the constructive principle of Nature applied to individual life."

"Disease is abnormal or inharmonious vibration of the elements and forces composing the human entity on one or more planes of being, in conformity with the destructive principle of Nature applied to individual life."

The question naturally arising here is, "Normal or abnormal vibration with what?" The answer is that the vibratory conditions of the organism must be in harmony with Nature's established harmonic relations in the physical, mental, moral, spiritual and psychical realms of human life and action.

What Is an Established Harmonic Relation?

Let us see whether we cannot make this clear by a simile. If a watch is in good condition, in harmonious vibration, its movement is so adjusted that it coincides exactly, in point of time, with the rotations of our earth around its axis. The established, regular movement of the earth forms the basis of the established harmonic relationship between the vibrations of a normal, healthy timepiece and the revolutions of our planet. The watch has to vibrate in unison with the harmonics of the planetary universe in order to be normal, or in harmony.

In like manner, everything that is normal, natural, healthy, good, beautiful must vibrate in unison with its correlated harmonics in Nature.

Obedience the Only Salvation

Orthodox medical science attributes disease largely to accidental causes: to chance infection by disease taints, germs or parasites; to drafts, chills, wet feet, etc.

The religiously inclined frequently attribute disease and other tribulations to the arbitrary rulings of an inscrutable Providence.

Christian Scientists tell us that sin, suffering, disease and all other kinds of evil are only errors of mortal mind, or the products of diseased imagination (though this in itself admits the existence of something abnormal or diseased).

Nature Cure philosophy presents a rational concept of evil, its cause and purpose, namely: that it is brought on by violation of Nature's Laws; that it is corrective in its purpose; that it can be overcome only by compliance with the law. There is no suffering, disease or evil of any kind anywhere unless the law has been transgressed somewhere by someone.

These transgressions of the law may be due to ignorance, to indifference or to wilfulness and viciousness. The effects will always be commensurate with the causes.

The science of natural living and healing shows clearly that what we call disease is primarily Nature's effort to eliminate morbid matter and to restore the normal functions of the body; that the processes of disease are just as orderly in their way as everything else in Nature; that we must not check or suppress them, but cooperate with them. Thus we learn, slowly and laboriously, the all-important lesson that "obedience to the law" is the only means of prevention of disease, and the only cure.

The Fundamental Law of Cure, the Law of Action and Reaction, and the Law of Crises, as revealed by the Nature Cure philosophy, impress upon us the truth that there is nothing accidental or arbitrary in the processes of health, disease and cure; that every changing condition is either in harmony or in discord with the laws of our being; that only by complete surrender and obedience to the law can we attain and maintain perfect physical health.

Self-Control, the Master's Key

Thus Nature Cure brings home to us constantly and forcibly the inexorable facts of natural law and the necessity of compliance with the law. Herein lies its great educational value to the individual and to the race. The man who has learned to master his habits and his appetites so as to conform to Nature's Laws on the physical plane, and who has thereby regained his bodily health, realizes that personal effort and self-control are the Master's Key to all further development on the mental and spiritual planes of being as well; that self-mastery and unremitting and unselfish personal effort are the only means of self-completion, of individual and social salvation.

The naturist who has regained health and strength through obedience to the laws of his being, enjoys a measure of self-content, gladness of soul and enthusiasm which cannot be explained by the mere possession of physical health. These highest and purest attainments of the human soul are not the results of mere physical well-being, but of the peace and harmony which come only from obedience to the law. Such is the peace which passeth understanding.

Chapter IV

The Unity of Disease and Treatment

There exists a close resemblance between the mechanism and the functions of a watch and of the human body. Their well-being is subject to similar underlying laws and principles. Both a watch and a human body may function abnormally as a result of accidental injury or unfavorable external conditions, such as extreme heat or cold, etc. However, in our present study of the causes of disease we shall not consider accidental injury and hostile environment, but confine ourselves to causes arising within the organism itself.

The watch may cease to vibrate in accord with the harmonics of our planetary universe for several reasons. It may lose time or stand still because (1) the wound spring has spent its force, or (2) its parts are not made up of the right constituents, or (3) foreign matter clogs or corrodes its mechanism.

Similarly, there exist three primary causes of disease and of premature death of the physical body. These are:

Lowered vitality. Abnormal composition of blood and lymph. Accumulation of morbid matter and poisons.

In the ultimate, disease and everything else that we designate as evil are the result of transgressions of natural laws in thinking, breathing, eating, dressing, working, resting, as well as in moral, sexual and social conduct.

In Tables I and II, I have endeavored to present in concise and comprehensive form the primary and the secondary causes or manifestations of disease and the corresponding natural methods of treatment.

TABLE I

~THE UNITY OF DISEASE AND TREATMENT~

Barring trauma (injury), advancing age and surroundings uncongenial to human life, all causes of disease may be classified as given below.

These established facts of greatly impaired longevity and universal abnormality of the human race would of themselves indicate that there is something radically wrong somewhere in the life habits of man, and that there is ample reason for the great health-reform movement which was started about the middle of the last century by the pioneers of Nature Cure in Germany, and which has since swept, under many different forms and guises, all portions of the civilized world.

When people in general grow better acquainted with the laws underlying prenatal and postnatal child culture, natural living and the natural treatment of diseases, human beings will approach much more closely the normal in health, strength, beauty and longevity. Then will arise a true aristocracy, not of morbid, venous blue blood, but pulsating with the rich red blood of health.

However, to reach this ideal of perfect physical, mental and moral health, succeeding generations will have to adhere to the natural ways of living and of treating their ailments. It cannot be attained by the present generation. The enthusiasts who claim that they can, by their particular methods, achieve perfect health and live the full term of human life, are destined to disappointment. We are so handicapped by the mistakes of the past that the best which most of us adults can do is to patch up, to attain a reasonable measure of health and to approach somewhat nearer Nature's full allotment of life.

Wild animals living in freedom retain their full vigor unimpaired almost to the end of life. Hunters report that among the great herds of buffalo, elk and deer, the oldest bucks are the rulers and maintain their sovereignty over the younger males of the herd solely by reason of their superior strength and prowess. Premature old age, among human beings, as indicated by the early decay of physical and mental powers, is brought on solely by their violation of Nature's Laws in almost all the ordinary habits of life.

Health Positive—Disease Negative

The freer the inflow of life force into the organism, the greater the vitality, the more there is of strength, of positive resisting and recuperating power.

In the book~ Harmonics of Evolution~ we are told that at the very foundation of the manifestation of life lies the principle of polarity, which expresses itself in the duality and unity of positive and negative affinity. The swaying to and fro of the positive and the negative, the desire to balance incomplete polarity, constitutes the very ebb and flow of life.

Disease is disturbed polarity. Exaggerated positive or negative conditions, whether physical, mental, moral or spiritual, tend to disease on the respective planes of being. Foods, medicines, suggestion and all the other different methods of therapeutic treatment exert on the individual subjected to them either a positive or a negative influence. It is, therefore, of the greatest importance that the physician and every one who wishes to live and work in harmony with Nature's Laws should understand this all-important question of magnetic polarity.

Lowered vitality means lowered, slower and coarser vibration, and this results in lowered resistance to the accumulation of morbid matter, poisons, disease taints, germs and parasites. This is what we designate ordinarily as the negative condition.

Let us see whether we can explain this more fully by a homely but practical illustration: A great many of my readers have probably seen in operation in the summer amusement parks the "human roulette." This contrivance consists of a large wheel, board-covered, somewhat raised in the center, and sloping towards the circumference. The wheel rotates horizontally, evenly with the floor or ground. The merrymakers pay their nickels for the privilege of throwing themselves flat down on the wheel and attempting to cling to it while it rotates with increasing swiftness. While the wheel moves slowly, it is easy enough to cling to it; but the faster it revolves, the more strongly the centrifugal force tends to throw off the human flies who try to stick to it.

The increasing repelling power of the accelerated motion of the wheel may serve as an illustration of that which we call vigorous vibration, good vitality, natural immunity or recuperative power. This is the positive condition.

The more intense the action of the life force, the more rapid and vigorous are the vibratory activities of the atoms and molecules in the cells, and of the cells in the organs and tissues of the body. The more rapid and vigorous this vibratory activity, the more powerful is the repulsion and expulsion of morbid matter, poisons and germs of disease which try to encumber or destroy the organism.

Health and Disease Resident in the Cell

We must not forget that health or disease, in the final analysis, is resident in the cell. Though a minute, microscopic organism, the cell is an independent living being, which is born, grows, eats, drinks, throws off waste matter, multiplies, ages and dies, just like man, the large cell. If the individual cell is well, man, the complex cell, is well also, and vice versa. From this it is apparent that in all our considerations of the processes of health, disease and cure, we have to deal primarily with the individual cell.

The vibratory activity of the cell may be lowered through the decline of vitality brought about in a natural way by advancing age, or in an artificial way through wrong habits of living, wrong thinking and feeling, overwork, unnatural stimulation and excesses of various kinds.

On the other hand, the inflow of vital force into the cells may be obstructed and their vibratory activity lowered by the accumulation of waste and morbid matter in the tissues, blood vessels and nerve channels of the body. Such clogging will interfere with the inflow of life force and with the free and harmonious vibration of the cells and organs of the body as surely as dust in a watch will interfere with the normal action and vibration of its wheels and balances.

From this it is evident that negative conditions may be brought about not only by hyperrefinement of the physical organism, but also by clogging it with waste and morbid matter which interfere with the inflow and distribution of the vital force. It also becomes apparent that in such cases the Nature Cure methods of eliminative treatment, such as pure food diet, hydrotherapy, massage, chiropractic, osteopathy, etc., are valuable means of removing these obstructions and promoting the inflow and free circulation of the positive electric and magnetic life currents

Abnormal Composition of Blood and Lymph

As one of the primary causes of disease, we cited abnormal composition of blood and lymph. The human organism is made up of a certain number of elements in well-defined proportions. Chem-istry has discovered, so far, about seventeen of these elements in appreciable quantities and has ascertained their functions in the economy of the body. These seventeen elements must be present in the right proportions in order to insure normal texture, structure and functioning of the component parts and organs of the body.

The cells and organs receive their nourishment from the blood and lymph currents. Therefore, these must contain all the elements needed by the organism in the right proportions, and this, of course, depends upon the character and the combination of the food supply.

Every disease arising in the human organism from internal causes is accompanied by a deficiency in blood and tissues of certain important mineral elements [organic salts]. Undoubtedly, the majority of these diseases are caused by an unbalanced diet, or by food and drink poisoning. Wrong food combinations, on the one hand, create an overabundance of waste and morbid matter in the system and, on the other hand, fail to supply the positive mineral elements or organic salts on which depends the elimination of waste and systemic poisons from the body.

The great problem of natural dietetics and of natural medical treatment is, therefore, how to restore and maintain the positivity of the blood and of the organism as a whole through providing in food, drink and medicine an abundant supply of the positive mineral salts in organic form.

Accumulation of Morbid Matter and Poisons

This is the third of the primary causes of disease. We have learned how lowered vitality and the abnormal composition of the vital fluids favor the retention of systemic poisons in the body. If, in addition to this, food and drink contain too much of the waste-producing carbohydrates, hydrocarbons and proteins, and not enough of the eliminating positive mineral salts then waste and morbid materials are bound to accumulate in the system and this results in the clogging of the tissues with acid precipitates and earthy deposits.

Such accumulation of waste and morbid matter in blood and tissues creates the great majority of all diseases arising within the human organism.

This will be explained fully in the following chapters which deal with the causation of acute and chronic disease.

More harmful and dangerous, and more difficult to eliminate than the different kinds of systemic poisons, that is, those which have originated within the body, are the drug poisons, especially when they are administered in the inorganic mineral form. Health is dependent upon an abundant supply of life force, upon the unobstructed, normal circulation of the vital fluids and upon perfect oxygenation and combustion. Anything that interferes with these essentials causes disease; anything that promotes them establishes health. Nothing so interferes with the inflow of the life force, with free and normal circulation of blood and lymph and with the oxygenation and combustion of food materials and systemic waste as the accumulation of morbid matter and poisons in the tissues of the body.

This I have endeavored to explain more fully in connection with lowered vitality. Let us now see how disease and health are affected by mental and emotional conditions.

Mental and Emotional Influences

Our mental and emotional conditions exert a most powerful influence upon the inflow and distribution of vital force. The author of The Great Work [~The Great Work: The Constructive Principle of Nature in Individual Life, ~by John Emmett Richardson {1853-1935}, Indio-American Book Company, Chicago, IL. 1907.] has described most graphically in the chapter on Self-Control how fear, worry, anxiety and all kindred emotions create in the system conditions similar to those of freezing; how these destructive vibrations congeal the tissues, clog the channels of life and paralyze the vital functions. He shows how the emotional conditions of impatience, irritability, anger, etc., have a heating, corroding effect upon the tissues of the body.

In like manner, all other destructive emotional vibrations obstruct the inflow and normal distribution of the life forces in and through the organism, while on the other hand the constructive emotions of faith, hope, cheerfulness, happiness and love exert a relaxing, harmonizing influence upon the tissues, blood vessels and nerve channels of the body, thus opening wide the floodgates of the life forces, and raising the discords of weakness, disease and discontent to the harmonics of buoyant health and happiness.

Let us see just how mind controls matter and how it affects the changing conditions of the physical body. Life manifests through vibration. It acts on the mass by acting through its minutest particles. Changes in the physical body are wrought by vibratory changes in atoms, molecules and cells. Health is satisfied polarity, that is, the balancing of the positive and negative elements in harmonious vibration. Anything that interferes with the free, vigorous and harmonious vibration of the minute parts and particles composing the human organism tends to disturb polarity and natural affinity, thus causing discord or disease.

When we fully realize these facts we shall not stand so much in awe of our physical bodies. In the past we have been thinking of the body as a solid and imponderable mass difficult to control and to change. This conception left us in a condition of utter helplessness and hopelessness in the presence of weakness and disease.

We now think of the body as composed of minute corpuscles rotating around one another within the atom at relatively immense distances. We know that in similar manner the atoms vibrate in the molecule, the molecules in the cell, the cells in the organ and the organs in the body; the whole capable of being changed by a change in the vibrations of its particles.

Thus the erstwhile solid physical mass appears plastic and fluidic, readily swayed and changed by the vibratory harmonies or discords of thoughts and emotions as well as by foods, medicines and therapeutic treatment.

Under the old conception the mind fell readily under the control of the body and became the abject slave of its physical conditions, swayed by fear and apprehension under every sensation of physical weakness, discomfort or pain. The servants lorded it with a high hand over the master of the house, and the result was chaos. Under the new conception, control is placed where it belongs. It is assumed by the real master of the house, the Soul-Man, and the servants, the physical members of the body, remain obedient to his bidding.

This is the new man, the ideal progeny of a new and higher philosophy. Understanding the structure of the body, the laws of its being and the operation of the life elements within it, the superman retains perfect poise and confidence under the most trying circumstances. Animated by an abounding faith in the supremacy of the healing forces within him and sustained by the power of his sovereign will, he governs his body as perfectly as the artist controls his violin and attunes its vibrations to Nature's harmonies of health and happiness.

Chapter V

The Unity of Acute Diseases

In the last chapter I endeavored to explain the three primary causes of disease, namely: (1) Lowered Vitality, (2) Abnormal Composition of Blood and Lymph, (3) Accumulation of Waste, Morbid Matter, and Poisons in the System.

We shall now consider some of the secondary manifestations resulting from these primary causes. Consulting the table on page 18 (Chapter 2, internet version), we find mentioned as the first one of the secondary causes or manifestations of disease, "Hereditary and Constitutional Taints."

On first impression, it might be thought that heredity is a primary cause of disease; but on further consideration it becomes apparent that it is an effect and not a primary cause. If the parents possess good vitality and pure, normal blood and tissues, and if they apply in the prenatal and postnatal treatment of the child the necessary insight and foresight, there cannot be disease heredity. In order to create abnormal hereditary tendencies, the parents, or earlier ancestors, must have ignorantly or wantonly violated Nature's Laws, such violation resulting in lowered vitality and in deterioration of blood and tissues.

The female and male germinal cells unite and form the primitive reproductive cell—the prototype of marriage. The human body with its millions of cells and cell colonies is developed by the multiplication, with gradual differentiation, of the reproductive cell. Its abnormalities of structure, of cell materials and of functional tendencies are reproduced just as surely as its normal constituents. Herein lies the simple explanation of heredity which is proved to be an actual fact, not only by common experience and scientific observation but also in a more definite way by Nature's records in the iris of the eye.

The iris of the newborn child reveals in its diagnostic details not only, in a general way, hereditary taints, lowered resistance, and deterioration of vital fluids, but frequently special weakness and deterioration in those organs which were weak or diseased in the parents. Under the conventional (unnatural) management of the infant, these hereditary tendencies to weakness and disease and their corresponding signs in the iris become more and more pronounced, proceeding through the various stages of incumbrance from acute, infantile diseases through chronic catarrhal conditions to the final destructive stages.

In the face of the well-established facts of disease heredity we have, however, this consolation: If the child be treated in accordance with the teachings of Nature Cure philosophy, the abnormal hereditary encumbrances and tendencies can be overcome and eliminated within a few years. If we place the infant organism under the right conditions of living and of treatment, in harmony with the laws of its being, the Life Principle within will approach ever nearer to the establishment of the perfect type. Hundreds of "Nature Cure" babies all over this country are living proofs of this gladsome message to all those who have assumed or intend to assume the responsibilities of parenthood.

Natural Immunity

Under Division II of "Secondary Causes or Manifestations of Disease" we find mentioned germs, bacteria, parasites, inflammations, fevers, skin eruptions, chronic sinus discharges, ulcers, etc.

Modern medical science is built up upon the germ theory of disease and treatment. Since the microscope has revealed the presence and seemingly entirely pernicious activity of certain microorganisms in connection with certain diseases, it has been assumed that bacteria are the direct, primary causes of most diseases. Therefore, the slogan now is: "Kill the bacteria (by poisonous antiseptics, serums and antitoxins) and you will cure the disease."

The Nature Cure philosophy takes a different view of the problem. Germs cannot be the cause of disease, because disease germs are also found in healthy bodies. The real cause must be something else. We claim that it is the waste and morbid matter in the system which afford the microorganisms of disease the opportunity to breed and multiply.

We regard microorganisms as secondary manifestations of disease, and maintain that bacteria and parasites live, thrive and multiply to the danger point in a weakened and diseased organism only. If it were not so, the human family would be extinct within a few months' time.

The fear instilled by the bacterial theory of disease is frequently more destructive than the microorganisms themselves. We have had under observation and treatment a number of insane patients whose peculiar delusion or monomania was an exaggerated fear of germs, a genuine bacteriophobia.

Keep yourself clean and vigorous from within, and you cannot be affected by disease taints and germs from without.

Bacteria are practically omnipresent. We absorb them in food and drink, we inhale them in the air we breathe. Our bodies are literally alive with them. The last stages of the digestive processes depend upon the activity of millions of bacteria in the intestinal tract.

The proper thing to do, therefore, is not to try and kill the germs, but to remove the morbid matter and disease taints in which they live.

Instead of concentrating its energies upon killing the germs, whose presence we cannot escape, Nature Cure endeavors to in-vigorate the system, to build up blood and lymph on a normal basis and to purify the tissues of their morbid encumbrances in such a way as to establish natural immunity to destructive germ activity. Everything that tends to accomplish this without injuring the system by poisonous drugs or surgical operations is good Nature Cure treatment.

To adopt the germ-killing process without purifying and invigorating the organism would be like trying to keep a house free from fungi and vermin by sprinkling it daily with carbolic acid and other germ killers, instead of keeping it pure and sweet by flooding it with fresh air and sunshine and applying freely and vigorously broom, brush and plenty of soap and water. Instead of purifying it, the antiseptics and germ killers would only add to the filth in the house.

All bacteriologists are unanimous in declaring that the various disease germs are found not only in the bodies of the sick, but also in seemingly healthy persons.

A celebrated French bacteriologist reports that in the mouth of a healthy infant, two months old, he found almost all the disease germs known to medical science. Only lately, a celebrated physician, appointed by the French government to investigate the causes of tuberculosis, declared before a meeting of the International Tuberculosis Congress in Rome that he found the bacilli of tuberculosis in ninety-five percent of all the school children he had examined.

Dr. Osler, one of the greatest living medical authorities, mentions repeatedly in his works that the bacilli of diphtheria, pneumonia and of many other virulent diseases are found in the bodies of healthy persons.

The inability of bacteria, by themselves, to create diseases is further confirmed by the well-known facts of natural immunity to specific infection or contagion. All mankind is more or less affected by hereditary and acquired disease taints, morbid encumbrances and drug poisoning, resulting from age-long violation of Nature's Laws and from the suppression of acute diseases; but even under the almost universal present conditions of lowered vitality, morbid heredity and physical and mental degeneration it is found that under identical conditions of exposure to drafts or infection, a certain percentage of individuals only will take the cold or catch the disease. The fact of natural immunity is constantly confirmed by common experience as well as in the clinics and laboratories of our medical schools and research institutes. Of a specific number of mice or rabbits inoculated with particles of cancer, only a small percentage develops the malignant growth and succumbs to its ravages.

The development of infectious and contagious diseases necessitates a certain predisposition, or, as medical science calls it, "disease diathesis." This predisposition to infection and contagion consists in the primary causes of disease, which we have designated as lowered vitality, abnormal composition of blood and lymph, and the accumulation of waste, morbid matter and poisons in the system.

Bacteria: Secondary, Not Primary,

Manifestations of Disease

In a previous chapter we learned how lowered vitality weakens the resistance of the system to the attacks and inroads of disease germs and poisons. The growth and multiplication of microorganisms depend furthermore upon a congenial, morbid soil. Just as the ordinary yeast germ multiplies in a sugar solution only, so the various microorganisms of disease thrive and multiply to the danger point only in their own peculiar and congenial kind of morbid matter. Thus, the typhoid fever bacillus thrives in a certain kind of effete matter which accumulates in the intestines; the pneumonia bacilli flourish best in the catarrhal secretions of the lungs, and meningitis bacilli in the diseased meninges of the brain and spinal cord.

Dr. Pettenkofer, a celebrated physician and professor of the University of Vienna, also arrived at the conclusion that bacteria, by themselves, cannot create disease, and for years he defended his opinion from the lecture platform and in his writings against the practically solid phalanx of the medical profession. One day he backed his theory by a practical test. While instructing his class in the bacteriological laboratory of the university, he picked up a glass which contained millions of live cholera germs and swallowed its contents before the eyes of the students. The seemingly dangerous experiment was followed only by a slight nausea. Lately I have heard repeatedly of persons in this country who subjected themselves in similar manner to infection, inoculation and contagion with the most virulent kinds of bacteria and disease taints without developing the corresponding diseases.

A few years ago Dr. Rodermund, a physician in the State of Wisconsin, created a sensation all over this country when he smeared his body with the exudate of smallpox sores in order to demonstrate to his medical colleagues that a healthy body could not be infected with the disease. He was arrested and quarantined in jail, but not before he had come in contact with many people. Neither he nor anyone else exposed by him developed smallpox.

During the ten years that I have been connected with sanitarium work, my workers and myself, in giving the various forms of manipulative treatment, have handled intimately thousands of cases of infectious and contagious diseases, and I do not remember a single instance where any one of us was in the least affected by such contact. Ordinary cleanliness, good vitality, clean blood and tissues, the organs of elimination in good, active condition and, last but not least, a positive, fearless attitude of mind will practically establish natural immunity to the inroads and ravages of bacteria and disease taints. If infection takes place, the organism reacts to it through inflammatory processes, and by means of these endeavors to overcome and eliminate microorganisms and poisons from the system.

In this connection it is of interest to learn that the danger to life from bites and stings of poisonous reptiles and insects has been greatly exaggerated. According to popular opinion, anyone bitten by a rattlesnake, gila monster or tarantula is doomed to die, while as a matter of fact the statistics show that only from two to seven per-cent succumb to the effects of the wounds inflicted by the bites of poisonous reptiles.

In this, as in many other instances, popular opinion should rather be called "popular superstition."

In the open discussions following my public lectures, I am often asked: "What is the right thing to do in case of snakebite? Would you not give plenty of whiskey to save the victim's life?"

It is my belief that of the seven percent who die after being bitten by rattlesnakes or other poisonous snakes, a goodly proportion give up the ghost because of the effects of the enormous doses of strong whiskey that are poured into them under the mistaken idea that the whiskey is an efficient antidote to the snake poison.

People do not know that the death rate from snakebite is so very low, and therefore they attribute the recoveries to the whiskey, just as recoveries from other diseases under medical or metaphysical treatment are attributed to the virtues of the particular medicine or method of treatment instead of to the real healer, the~ vis medicatrix nature,~ the healing power of Nature, which in ninety-three cases in a hundred eliminates the rattlesnake venom without injury to the organism.

To recapitulate: Just as yeast cells are not only the cause but also the product of sugar fermentation, so disease germs are not only a cause (secondary) but also a product of morbid fermentation in the system. Furthermore, just as yeast germs live on and decompose sugar, so disease germs live on and decompose morbid matter and systemic poisons.

In a way, therefore, microorganisms are just as much the product as the cause of disease and act as scavengers or eliminators of morbid matter. In order to hold in check the destructive activity of bacteria and to prevent their multiplication beyond the danger point, Nature resorts to inflammation and manufactures her own antitoxins.

On the other hand, whatever tends to build up the blood on a natural basis, to promote elimination of morbid matter and thereby to limit the activity of destructive microorganisms without injuring the body or depressing its vital functions, is good Nature Cure practice. The first consideration, therefore, in the treatment of inflammation must be to not interfere with its natural course.

By the various statements and claims made in this chapter, I do not wish to convey the idea that I am opposed to scrupulous cleanliness or surgical asepsis. Far from it! These are dictates of common sense. But I do affirm that the danger from germ and other infectious diseases lies just as much or more so in internal filth as in external uncleanliness. Cleanliness and asepsis must go hand in hand with the purification of the inner man in order to insure natural immunity.

Chapter VI

The Laws of Cure

This brings us to the consideration of acute inflammatory and feverish diseases. From what has been said, it follows that inflammation and fever are not primary, but secondary, manifestations of disease. There cannot arise any form of inflammatory disease in the system unless there is present some enemy to health which Nature is endeavoring to overcome and get rid of. On this fact in Nature is based what I claim to be the fundamental Law of Cure.

"Give me fever and I can cure every disease." Thus Hippocrates the Father of Medicine, expressed the fundamental Law of Cure over two thousand years ago. I have expressed this law in the following sentence: "Every acute disease is the result of a cleansing and healing effort of Nature."

This law, when thoroughly understood and applied to the treatment of diseases, will in time do for medical science what the discovery of other natural laws has done for physics, astronomy, chemistry and other exact sciences. It will transform the medical empiricism and confusion of the past and present into an exact science by demonstrating the unity of disease and treatment.

Applying the law in a general way, it means that all acute diseases, from a simple cold to measles, scarlet fever, diphtheria, smallpox, pneumonia, etc., represent Nature's efforts to repair injury or to remove from the system some kind of morbid matter, virus, poison or microorganism dangerous to health and life. In other words, acute diseases cannot develop in a perfectly normal, healthy body living under conditions favorable to human life. The question may be asked: "If acute diseases represent Nature's healing efforts, why is it that people die from them?" The answer to this is: the vitality may be too low, the injury or morbid encumbrance too great or the treatment may be inadequate or harmful, so that Nature loses the fight; still, the acute disease represents an effort of Nature to overcome the enemies to health and life and to reestablish normal, healthy conditions.

It is a curious fact that this fundamental principle of Nature Cure and Law of Nature has been acknowledged and verified by medical science. The most advanced works on pathology admit the constructive and beneficial character of inflammation. However, when it comes to the treatment of acute diseases, physicians seem to forget entirely this basic principle of pathology, and treat inflammation and fever as though they were, in themselves, inimical and destructive to health and life.

From this inconsistency in theory and practice arise all the errors of allopathic medical treatment. Failure to understand this fundamental Law of Cure accounts for all the confusion on the part of the exponents of the different schools of healing sciences, and for the greater part of human suffering.

The Nature Cure philosophy never loses sight of the fundamental Law of Cure. While allopathy regards acute disease conditions as in themselves harmful and hostile to health and life, as something to be cured (we should say suppressed) by drug or knife, the Nature Cure school regards these forcible housecleanings as beneficial and necessary, so long, at least, as people will continue to disregard Nature's Laws. While, through its simple, natural methods of treatment, Nature Cure easily modifies the course of inflammatory and feverish processes and keeps them within safe limits, it never checks or suppresses these acute reactions by poisonous drugs, serums, antiseptics, surgical operations, suggestion or any other suppressive treatment.

Skin eruptions, boils, ulcers, catarrhs, diarrheas, and all other forms of inflammatory febrile disease conditions are indications that there is something hostile to life and health in the organism which Nature is trying to remove or overcome by these so-called "acute" diseases. What, then, can be gained by suppressing them with poisonous drugs and surgical operations? Such practice does not allow Nature to carry on her work of cleansing and repair and to attain her ends. The morbid matter which she endeavored to eliminate by acute reactions is thrown back into the system. Worse than that, drug poisons are added to disease poisons. Is it any wonder that fatal complications arise, or that the acute condition is changed to chronic disease?

Why Does the Greater Part of Allopathic Materia

Medica Consist of Virulent Poisons?

The statements made in the preceding pages are a severe indictment of regular medical science, but they point out the difference in the basic principles of the "Old School" of healing and those of the Nature Cure philosophy.

The fundamental Law of Cure quoted in this chapter explains why allopathic medical science is in error, not in a few things only, but in most things. The foundation, the orthodox conception of disease being wrong, it follows that everything which is built thereon must be wrong also.

No matter how learned a man may be, if he begins a problem in arithmetic with the proposition 2x2=5, he never will arrive at a correct solution if he continue to figure into all eternity. Neither can allopathy solve the problem of disease and cure as long as its fundamental conception of disease is based on error.

The fundamental law of cure explains also why the great majority of allopathic prescriptions contain virulent poisons in some form or another and why surgical operations are in high favor with the disciples of the regular school.

The answer of allopathy to the question, "Why do you give poisons?" usually is, "Our materia medica contains poisons because drug poison kills and eliminates disease poison." We, however, claim that drug poisons merely serve to paralyze vital force, whereby the deceptive results of allopathic treatment are obtained.

The following will explain this more fully. We have learned that so-called acute diseases are Nature's cleansing and healing efforts. All acute reactions represent increased activity of vital force, resulting in feverish and inflammatory conditions, accompanied by pain, redness, swelling, high temperature, rapid pulse, catarrhal discharges, skin eruptions, boils, ulcers, etc.

Allopathy regards these violent activities of vital force as detrimental and harmful in themselves. Anything which will inhibit the action of vital force will, in allopathic parlance, cure (?) acute diseases. As a matter of fact, nothing more effectively paralyzes vital force and impairs the vital organs than poisonous drugs and the surgeon's knife. These, therefore, must necessarily constitute the favorite means of cure (?) of the regular school of medicine.

This school mistakes effect for cause. It fails to see that the local inflammation arising within the organism is not the disease, but merely marks the locality and the method through which Nature is trying her best to discharge the morbid encumbrances; that the acute reaction is local, but that its causes or feeders are always constitutional and must be treated constitutionally. When, under the influence of rational, natural treatment, the poisonous irritants are eliminated from blood and tissues, the local symptoms take care of themselves; it does not matter whether they manifest as pimple or cancer, as a simple cold or as consumption.

The Law of Dual Effect

Everywhere in Nature rules the great Law of Action and Reaction. All life sways back and forth between giving and receiving, between action and reaction. The very breath of life mysteriously comes and goes in rhythmical flow. So also heaves and falls in ebb and tide the bosom of Mother Earth.

In some of its aspects, this law is called the Law of Compensation, or the Law of Dual Effect. On its action depends the preservation of energy.

The Great Master expressed the ethical application of this law when he said:

"Give, and it shall be given unto you. . . . For with the same measure that ye mete it shall be measured to you again."—Luke 6:38.

In the realms of physical nature, giving and receiving, action and reaction balance each other mechanically and automatically. What we gain in power we lose in speed or volume, and vice versa. This makes it possible for the mechanic, the scientist and the astronomer to predict with mathematical precision for ages in advance the results of certain activities in Nature.

The great Law of Dual Effect forms the foundation of the healing sciences. It is related to and governs every phenomenon of health, disease and cure. When I formulated the fundamental Law of Cure in the words, "Every acute disease is the result of a healing effort of Nature," this was but another expression of the great Law of Action and Reaction. What we commonly call crisis, acute reaction or acute disease is in reality Nature's attempt to establish health.

Applied to the physical activity of the body, the Law of Com-pensation may be expressed as follows: "Every agent affecting the human organism produces two effects: a first, apparent, temporary effect, and a second, lasting effect. The secondary, lasting effect is always contrary to the primary, transient effect."

For instance: The first and temporary effect of cold water applied to the skin consists in sending the blood to the interior; but in order to compensate for the local depletion, Nature responds by sending greater quantities of blood back to the surface, resulting in increased warmth and better surface circulation.

The first effect of a hot bath is to draw the blood to the surface; but the secondary effect sends the blood back to the interior, leaving the surface bloodless and chilled.

Stimulants, as we shall see later on, produce their deceptive effects by burning up the reserve stores of vital energy in the organism. This is inevitably followed by weakness and exhaustion in exact proportion to the previous excitation.

The primary effect of relaxation and sleep is weakness, numbness and death-like stupor; the secondary effect, however, is an increase of vitality.

The Law of Dual Effect governs all drug action. The first, temporary, violent effect of poisonous drugs, when given in physiological doses, is usually due to Nature's efforts to overcome and eliminate these substances. The secondary, lasting effect is due to the retention of the drug poisons in the system and their action on the organism.

In theory and practice, allopathy considers the first effect only and ignores the lasting aftereffects of drugs and surgical operations. It administers remedies whose first effect is contrary to the disease condition. Therefore, in accordance with the Law of Action and Reaction, the secondary, lasting effect of such remedies must be similar to or like the disease condition.

Common, everyday experience should teach us that this is so, for laxatives and cathartics always tend to produce chronic constipation.

The secondary effect of stimulants and tonics of any kind is increased weakness, and their continued use often results in complete exhaustion and paralysis of mental and physical powers.

Headache powders, pain killers, opiates, sedatives and hypnotics may paralyze brain and nerves into temporary insensibility; but, if due to constitutional causes, the pain, nervousness and insomnia will always return with redoubled force. If taken habitually, these agents invariably tend to create heart disease and paralysis, and ultimately develop the patient into a dope fiend.

Cold and catarrh cures (?), such as quinine, coal-tar products, etc., suppress Nature's efforts to eliminate waste and morbid matter through the mucous linings of the respiratory tract, and drive the disease matter back into the lungs, thus breeding pneumonia, chronic catarrhs, asthma and consumption.

Mercury, iodine and all other alteratives, by suppression of external elimination, create internal chronic diseases of the most dreadful types, such as locomotor ataxy, paresis, etc.

So the recital might be continued all through orthodox materia medica. Each drug breeds new disease symptoms which are in their turn cured (?) by other poisons, until the insane asylum or merciful death rings down the curtain on the tragedy of a ruined life.

The teaching and practice of homeopathy, as explained in Chapter Twenty-Six, is fully in harmony with the Law of Action and Reaction. Acting upon the basic principle of homeopathy: ~Similia similibus curantur,~ or like cures like, it administers remedies whose first, temporary effect is similar to the disease conditions. In accordance with the Law of Dual Effect, then, the secondary effect of these remedies must be contrary to the disease conditions, that is, curative.

Chapter VII

Suppression Versus Elimination

My claim that the conventional treatment of acute diseases is suppressive and not curative will probably be denied by my medical colleagues. They will maintain that their methods also are calculated to eliminate morbid matter and disease germs from the system.

But what are the facts in actual practice? Is it not true that preparations of mercury, lead, zinc and other powerful poisons are constantly used to suppress skin eruptions, boils, abscesses, etc., instead of allowing Nature to rid the system through these skin diseases of scrofulous, venereal and psoric taints?

Some time ago Dr. Wiley, the former Government Chemist, published the ingredients of a number of popular remedies for colds, coughs and catarrh. Every one of them contained some powerful opiate or astringent. These poisonous drugs relieve the cough and the catarrhal conditions by paralyzing the eliminative activity of the membranous linings of the nasal passages, the bronchi and lungs, the digestive and genitourinary organs; but in doing so, they throw back into the system the morbid matter which Nature is trying to get rid of, and add drug poisons to disease poisons.

Equally harmful is suppression by means of the surgeon's knife. It may be a quicker and apparently more effective process to remove the inflamed appendix or the diseased tonsils than to cure them by building up the blood and inducing elimination of systemic poisons by natural methods. But operative treatment is not eliminative. It does not remove from the system the original cause of the inflammation or deterioration of tissues and organs, but it does remove the outlet which Nature had established for the escape of morbid materials.

These morbid encumbrances, forcibly retained in the body, weaken and destroy other parts and organs, or affect the general health of the patient.

My own observations during nearly fifteen years of practical experience, confirmed by many other conscientious observers among Nature Cure practitioners as well as physicians of other schools and of allopathy itself, prove positively that the average length of life after a major operation, performed on important, vital parts and organs, is less than ten years, and that after such an operation the general health of the patient is in the great majority of cases not as good as before.

In the following paragraphs are mentioned some very common instances of suppression and some of their usual chronic aftereffects (sequelae).

Diarrhea is suppressed with laudanum and other opiates, which paralyze the peristaltic action of the bowels and, if repeated, soon produce chronic constipation. Gonorrheal discharges and syphilitic ulcers are checked and suppressed by local injections, cauterization and by prescriptions containing mercury, iodine and other poisonous alternatives which effectually prevent Nature's efforts to eliminate the venereal poisons from the system.

Gonorrheal discharges and syphilitic ulcers are checked and supressed by local injections, cauterizatin, and by prescriptions containing mercury, iodine, and other poisonous alternatives which effectually prevent Nature's efforts to elminate the venereal poisons from the system.

All feverish diseases are more or less interfered with or suppressed by antiseptics, antipyretics, serums and antitoxins. The best books on ~Materia Medica~ and the professors in the colleges teach that these remedies lower the fever because they are "protoplasmic poisons"; because they paralyze the red and white blood corpuscles, benumb heart action and respiration, and depress all vital functions.

Nervousness, sleeplessness and pain are suppressed by sedatives, opiates and hypnotics. Every one of the drugs used for such purposes is a powerful poison which paralyzes brain and nerve action, in that way interfering with Nature's healing efforts and frequently preventing the consummation of beneficial healing crises.

Epileptic attacks and other forms of convulsions are suppressed, but never cured, by bromides which benumb and paralyze the brain and nerve centers. All that these sedatives accomplish is to produce in the course of time idiocy and the different forms of paralysis and premature senility.

However, is he not considered the best doctor who can most promptly produce these and many similar deceptive results through artificial inhibition or stimulation by means of the most virulent poisons found on earth?

Dandruff and falling hair are caused by the elimination of systemic poisons through the scalp. The thing to do, therefore, is not to suppress this elimination and thereby cause the accumulation of poisons in the brain, but to stop the manufacture of poison in the body and to promote its removal through the natural channels.

Dandruff cures and hair tonics contain glycerine, poisonous antiseptics and stimulants which are absorbed by scalp and brain, causing dizziness, headaches, loss of memory, neurasthenia, deaf-ness, weakness of sight, etc.

Head lice and similar parasites peculiar to other parts of the body live on scrofulous and psoriotic taints. When these are consumed, the lice depart as they came, no one knows whence or whither.

This is confirmed by the fact that these noxious pests do not remain with all people who have been exposed to them, but only with those whose internal or external filth conditions furnish the parasites with the means of subsistence.

In a number of instances we have seen "healing crises" take the form of lice. At that time the patients were living in the most clean surroundings, taking different forms of water treatment every day and infection was practically impossible.

These people invariably recalled that they had been infested with parasites at some previous time, and that strong antiseptics, mercurial salves, or other means of suppression had been applied.

We prescribe for the removal of lice only cold water and the comb. Even antiseptic soaps should be avoided.

The Results of Suppression of Children's Diseases

Sycotic eruptions on the heads and bodies of infants, also called milk scurf, if suppressed by salves, cream, unsalted butter or merely by warm bathing, are often followed by chorea (St. Vitus' dance), epilepsy, a scrofulous constitution and in later life by tuberculosis.

Measles, scarlet fever, diphtheria, spinal meningitis and other febrile diseases of childhood, if properly treated by natural methods, are curative or at least corrective in their effects on the system, and represent well-defined, orderly natural processes for the elimination of inherited or acquired disease taints, drug poisons, etc. But if arrested or suppressed before they have run their natural course, before Nature has had time to reestablish normal conditions, then the abnormal condition becomes fixed and permanent (chronic).

In addition to this, the poisons and serums employed to arrest the disease process very often affect vital parts and organs permanently, causing the gradual deterioration of cells and tissues, and paving the way for tuberculosis, chronic affection of the kidneys, cancer, etc., in later years.

These self-evident facts, which can be verified by any unprejudiced observer, account for the "mysterious sequelae" of drug-and serum-treated acute diseases, which never occur where natural methods of healing have been correctly employed. Some of these chronic aftereffects are deafness, blindness, heart and kidney diseases, nervous affections, idiocy, infantile paralysis, etc.

These are merely a few ordinary examples of the results of suppression. They could be multiplied a hundred fold, yet medical science assures us that the causes of cancer and other malignant diseases are unknown.

Good Nature Cure Doctrine from an Allopathic Authority

The following utterances of the late Dr. Nicholas Senin strongly confirm our claims as to the nature and cure of disease. Coming from the lips of a celebrated surgeon and physician, these statements should carry some weight with those who, being unable to reason for themselves, worship at the feet of "authority." The quotations referred to are taken from the report of an interview granted by the doctor to Chicago newspaper representatives on his return from his trip around the world.

[Chicago American, August 5th, 1906.]

GERMS PLANTED BY TIGHT LACING

Over-Feeding and Over-Dressing Given as Causes of Cancer

"Dr. Nicholas Senn brought back from Africa, from whence he returned to Chicago yesterday, confirmations of his belief that cancer is a 'civilized' disease.

"Dr. Senn spent from $2,000 to $3,000 worth of time—at the cash value per hour of his time on his first day at home for four months, telling a half dozen newspaper men more than all the world, except himself and a score of specialists like him, know about the fearful disease. He summed up his own learning in the statement that the disease is still incurable except by the knife in its incipient stages and that the best preventive is clean, plain living.

"His investigations of the natives of Africa served to strengthen his conviction that cancer is a product of civilization, 'like apoplexy and scores of other exotic ailments,' Dr. Senn said. He could not find or hear of a case of cancer among the 'Hamites,' as he termed them. And from the fact that he found the disease, to be an unknown one to the Esquimaux of Greenland, he is assured that climate has nothing whatever to do with it. Climate did not cause it, and climate will not cure it."

Cancer Caused by Over-Living

"'The nearer the human race approaches the animals in habits and particularly in the matter of diet and dress, the freer it is from cancer,' he said. 'Cancer comes from over-feeding and over-living.

"'Drinking, gourmandizing, unnatural habits of women, like lacing, all those things help to plant the seeds of cancer in the child.

"'And as we have not learned to cure it the best thing to do is to prevent it when we can. If children were brought up in simplicity by natural mothers; then, if care should be taken to prevent hypernutrition, there would be much less danger from cancer. Cancer itself is an over-fed thing—tissue that never matures, for if I could mature the cells I could cure the disease. The thing for people to do who fear they may have inherited it, is to live simply —there are many cases among people with a tendency to obesity to one among those of a scanty habit of living—and particularly to remove all sources of irritation, like bad teeth, tobacco, and clothes that chafe.'"

Studies African Race

"Besides his hobby, as he calls it, Dr. Senn studied the African generally in his voyage along the East Coast of that continent.

"'It was a fine trip,' he said, 'with so many things to learn. Ethnologically I am certain Africans are of common stock. The negro is a negro wherever you find him. From Kaffir to Bushman and pygmy they are all Hamites.

"'They are mostly a fine people physically, lean and tall, except the dwarfs. There is little tendency toward obesity; they have no apoplexy, no distended veins as we have in civilization. Hence their freedom from cancer. They live naturally, and are vegetarians mostly, while the Northern Esquimaux are meat-eaters, but both races eat naturally to sustain life, hence their immunity from that disease. It is where eating is made an art that cancer is most prevalent.

"'They are free from many other diseases that pester us also. Tuberculosis is hardly known, and only along the coast, where it has been taken by the whites. The real curse of the coast country is malaria. It is bad all up and down the East shore. I kept away from it myself by taking five grains of quinine and the juice of a lemon once a day on an empty stomach. That is a good remedy for malaria, for in all my running around I have never had it."

(Editor's Note.—Dr. Senn died January 2, 1908. The papers stated after his death, that the doctor had never been well since the return from his long voyage, that his heart and nervous system had been seriously affected by the altitudes of the Andes and of other mountains. We wonder whether the "high altitudes" or the "five grains of quinine daily" were to blame for the celebrated physician's heart disease and death.)

Suppression, the Cause of Chronic Diseases

Dr. Senn was right. If men and women lived more naturally, the majority of diseases would disappear.

The primary cause of disease is violation of Nature's Laws. "Civilization" has largely stood for artificiality of life and for unnatural habits. A higher civilization, yet to come, will combine the most exquisite culture of heart and mind with true simplicity and naturalness of living. Excessive meat eating, strong spices and condiments, alcohol, coffee, tea, overwork, night work, fear, worry, sensuality, corsets, high heels, foul air, improper breathing, lack of exercise, loveless marriages, race suicide, all of these and many other evils of hypercivlization have contributed their share in creating the universal degeneracy of civilized nations commented upon by Dr. Senn.

When the unnatural habits of life alluded to have lowered the vitality and favored the accumulation of waste matter and poisons to such an extent that the sluggish bowels, kidneys, skin and the other organs of elimination are unable to keep a clean house, Nature has to resort to other, more radical means of purification or we should choke in our own impurities. These forcible housecleanings of Nature are colds, catarrh, skin eruptions, diarrheas, boils, ulcers, abnormal perspiration, hemorrhages and many other forms of inflammatory febrile diseases.

Sulphur and mercury may drive back the skin eruptions, antipyretics and antiseptics may suppress fever and catarrh. The patient and the doctor may congratulate themselves on a speedy cure; but what is the true state of affairs? Nature has been thwarted in her work of healing and cleansing. She had to give up the fight against disease matter in order to combat the more potent poisons of mercury, quinine, iodine, strychnine, etc. The disease matter is still in the system, plus the drug poison.

Proof positive of the retention of drug poisons in the organism is furnished by the Diagnosis from the Eye. This will be explained more fully in another chapter.

When vitality has been sufficiently restored, Nature may make another attempt at purification, this time, possibly, in another direction; but again her well-meant efforts are defeated. This process of suppression is repeated over and over again until blood and tissues become so loaded with waste material and poisons that the healing forces of the organism can no longer react against them by acute diseases. Then results the chronic condition, which in the vocabulary of the "Old School" of medicine is only another name for incurable disease.

The more skilled the allopathic school becomes in the suppression and prevention of acute diseases by drugs, knife, x-rays, serums, vaccination virus, etc., the greater will be the increase of chronic dyspepsia, nervous prostration, insanity, locomotor ataxy, paresis, cancer, secondary and tertiary syphilis, tuberculosis and many other so-called incurable diseases. Thus, the standard medical practice is self-supporting; the treatment of acute conditions assuring a lifelong supply of chronic conditions for the doctor to treat.

Suppression of acute diseases, by drugs and knife, is the all-important factor in the creation of malignant diseases which Dr. Senn had overlooked in his discourse on the causes of distructive ailments. If he had steudied his experiences in foreign lands in the light of these explanations he would have found that these scourges of mankind exist only in those parts of earth where the drug store flourishes.

These statements may seem exaggerated; but allow me to cite a few typical cases of suppression and their effects upon the system from our daily practice.

Paresis, locomotor ataxy and paralysis agitans are not, as is usually assumed, due to secondary and tertiary syphilis, but to the mercury administered for the cure of luetic and other diseases. In less than six months' time we cure the so-called specific diseases by our natural methods, provided they are not suppressed and complicated by mercury, iodine or other poisonous drugs. We never interfere with the original lesion, but allow Nature to discharge the poisons through the channels established for this purpose.

Under this rational treatment, discharge and ulcer act as fontanels to the system. Not only the specific poison, but much of hereditary and acquired disease matter also are eliminated in the process; and after such a cure, blood and tissues of the patient are purer than they were before infection.

The foregoing statement has nothing to do with the moral aspects involved in acquiring venereal diseases. In this connection we are dealing solely with the rational or irrational treatment of the infection after it has been contracted. We do not wish to intimate that it is advisable to cure the body by killing the soul.

Nevertheless, we must deal with the facts in Nature as we find them. Furthermore, a great many persons, especially women and children, acquire these diseases innocently. Are we not justified in relieving their minds of needless fear and in showing them the way to prevent the dreadful sufferings of the secondary and tertiary stages brought on by suppressive drug treatment by means of mercury, the iodides, "606," etc.?

These poisonous drugs suppress the initial lesion and diffuse the disease poison through the system. Nature takes up the work of elimination by means of skin eruptions and ulcers in various parts of the body, but these also are promptly suppressed with mercurial ointments and other alternatives. This process of suppression is continued for months and years, until the organism is so thoroughly saturated with alterative poisons that vital force can no longer react by acute reactions against the original syphilitic poisons. This state of vital paralysis is then called a cure.

The medical professor, however, knows better. He instructs the students from the lecture platform: "When, after two or three years of mercurial treatment, syphilitic symptoms cease to appear, you may permit the patient to marry—but never guarantee a cure."

Why not? Because the professor is aware that the offspring of such a union are born with hereditary symptoms well known to every physician, and because the patient thus cured (?) may turn up in the doctor's office at any time thereafter with a hole in his palate, ulcers on his body, caries of the bones or with other secondary and tertiary symptoms.

Mercury has an especial affinity for the bony structures. It will work its way through the vertebrae of the spine and the bones of the skull into the nerve matter of the brain and spinal cord, causing inflammation, excruciating headaches, nervous symptoms, girdle pains, etc. These stages of acute inflammation are followed in a few years by sclerosis (hardening) of nerve matter and blood vessels, resulting in paresis, locomotor ataxy or paralysis agitans.

Neither is it necessary to contract specific diseases in order to fall a victim to these dreadful conditions: mercury, iodine and other destructive alternatives are given in a hundred different forms for a multitude of other ailments.

A few years ago we had under our care a patient in the last stages of locomotor ataxy, who for years had been suffering the tortures of the damned. There had never been a taint of specific disease in her system, but four different times in her life she had been salivated by calomel (a common laxative containing mercury). This dreadful poison was given to her in large doses for the cure of liver trouble and constipation. She was only fourteen years old when, on account of this, she first suffered from acute mercurial poisoning.

Another patient who, after fifteen years of slow and torturous dying by inches, succumbed to the same disease, absorbed the mercurial poison in his boyhood days while attending a boarding school. He was twice salivated by mercurial ointments applied to cure the itch (scabies), a disease which was epidemic at times among the boys. He likewise never had a syphilitic disease.

A young man, insane at the age of thirty, absorbed the infernal poison when four years of age. He had at the time a psoric skin eruption, but the family physician suspected syphilitic infection from the nurse girl and kept the child under mercury for six months. How do we know that the diagnosis of syphilis was false? Because the iris of the eye revealed "psora" as the cause of the suspicious eruption which reappeared several times later in life, and because the servant girl was afterwards absolutely exonerated by competent physicians.

Proofs by the Diagnosis from the Eye

We have treated many hundreds of cases of so-called chronic neuralgia, neuritis, rheumatism, neurasthenia, epilepsy and idiocy, due to the pernicious effects of quinine, iodine, arsenic, strychnine, coal-tar products and other virulent poisons taken under the guise of medicine.

How do we know that this is so?

Because the Diagnosis from the Eye plainly reveals the presence of these poisons in the system. Because the drug signs in the eye are accompanied by the symptoms of these poisons in the system. Because the record in the eye is confirmed by the history of the patient. Because, under natural living and treatment, diseases long ago suppressed by drugs or knife reappear as healing crises. Because, in these healing crises, drugs indicated by the signs in the iris of the eye are frequently eliminated under their own peculiar symptoms. Because, to the extent that a drug is eliminated from the system by a healing crisis, its sign will disappear from the iris of the eye.

To illustrate:

The Diagnosis from the Eye reveals heavy quinine poisoning in the region of the brain. This enables us to say to the patient, without questioning him, that he suffers from severe frontal headaches and ringing in the ears, that he is very irritahle, and so on through the various symptoms of quinine poisoning. The history of the patient reveals the fact that he has taken large amounts of quinine for colds, la grippe or malaria. Under our methods of natural living and treatment, the patient improves; the organism becomes more vigorous, and the organs of elimination act more freely; the latent poisons are stirred up in their hiding places; healing crises make their appearance. The processes of elimination thus inaugurated develop various symptoms of acute poisoning. The eliminating crises are accompanied by headaches, ringing in the ears, nasal catarrh, bone pains, neuritis, strong taste of quinine in the mouth, etc. Every healing crisis, if naturally treated, diminishes the signs of disease and drug poisons in the eye.

Chapter VIII

Inflammation

From what has already been said on this subject, it will have become apparent that inflammatory and feverish diseases are just as natural, orderly and lawful as anything else in Nature, that, therefore, after they have once started, they must not be checked or suppressed by poisonous drugs and surgical operations.

Inflammatory processes can be kept within safe limits, and they must be assisted in their constructive tendencies by the natural methods of treatment. To check and suppress acute diseases before they have run their natural course means to suppress Nature's purifying and healing efforts, to court fatal complications and to change the acute, constructive reactions into chronic disease conditions.

Those who have followed the preceding chapters will remember that their general trend has been to prove one of the fundamental principles of Nature Cure philosophy, namely the Unity of Disease and Cure.

We claim that all acute diseases are uniform in their causes, their purpose, and if conditions are favorable, uniform also in their progressive development.

In former chapters I endeavored to prove and to elucidate the unity of acute diseases in regard to their causes and their purpose, the latter not being destructive, but constructive and beneficial. I demonstrated that the microorganisms of disease are not the unmitigated nuisance and evil which they are commonly regarded, but that, like everything else in Nature, they, too, serve a useful purpose. I showed that it depends upon ourselves whether their activity is harmful and destructive, or beneficial: upon our manner of living and of treating acute reactions.

Let us now trace the unity of acute diseases in regard to their general course by a brief examination of the processes of inflammation and their progressive development through five well-defined stages. We shall base our studies on the most advanced works on pathology and bacteriology.

The Story of Inflammation

The organism has still other ways and means of defending itself. At the time of bacterial infection, certain germ-killing substances are developed in the blood serum. Science has named these defensive proteins ~alexins.~ It has also been found that the phagocyte and tissue cells in the neighborhood of the area of irritation produce antipoisons or natural antitoxins, which neutralize the bacterial poisons and kill the microorganisms of disease.

With the Evil, Nature Provides the Cure

Furthermore, the growth and development of bacteria and parasites is inhibited and finally arrested by their own waste products. We have an example of this in the yeast germ, which thrives and multiplies in the presence of sugar in solution. Living on and digesting the sugar, it decomposes the sugar molecules into alcohol and carbonic acid. As the alcohol increases during the process of fermentation, it gradually arrests the development and activity of the yeast cells.

Similar phenomena accompany the activity of disease germs and parasites. They produce certain waste products which gradually inhibit their own growth and increase. The vaccines, serums and antitoxins of medical science are prepared from these bacterial excrements and from extracts made of the bodies of bacteria.

In the serum and antitoxin treatment, therefore, the allopathic school is imitating Nature's procedure in checking the growth of microorganisms, but with this difference: Nature does not suppress the growth and multiplication of disease germs until the morbid matter on which they subsist has been decomposed and consumed, and until the inflammatory processes have run their course through the five stages of inflammation; while serums and antitoxins given in powerful doses at the different stages of any disease may check and suppress germ activity and the processes of inflammation before the latter have run their natural course and before the morbid matter has been eliminated.

The Five Stages of Inflammation

What has been said in former chapters confirms my claim that all acute diseases are uniform in their causes and in their purpose. From the foregoing description of inflammation it will have become clear that they are also uniform in their pathological development. The uniformity of acute inflammatory processes becomes still more apparent when we follow them through their five succeeding stages, that is: Incubation, Aggravation, Destruction, Abatement and Reconstruction, as illustrated in the following diagram:

I. Incubation. The first section of the diagram corresponds to the period of Incubation, the time between the exposure to an infectious disease and its development. This period may last from a few minutes to a few days, weeks, months or even years.

During this stage morbid matter, poisons, microorganisms and other excitants of inflammation gather and concentrate in certain parts and organs of the body. When they have accumulated to such an extent as to interfere with the normal functions or to endanger the health and life of the organism, the life forces begin to react to the obstruction or threatening danger by means of the inflammatory processes before described.

II. Aggravation. During the period of Aggravation the battle between the phagocytes and Nature's antitoxins on the one hand, and the poisons and microorganisms of disease on the other hand, gradually progresses, accompanied by a corresponding increase of fever and inflammation, until it reaches its climax, marked by the greatest intensity of feverish symptoms.

III. Destruction. This battle between the forces of disease and the healing forces is accompanied by the disintegration of tissues due to the accumulation of exudates, to pus formation, the development of abscesses, boils, fistulas, open sores, etc., and to other morbid changes. It involves the destruction of phagocytes, bacteria, blood vessels, and tissues just as a battle between contending human armies results in loss of life and property.

The stage of Destruction ends in crisis, which may be either fatal or beneficial. If the healing forces of the organism are in the ascendancy, and if they are supported by right treatment which tends to build up the blood, increase the vitality and promote elimination, then the poisons and the microorganisms of disease will gradually be overcome, absorbed or eliminated and, by degrees, the tissues will be cleared of the debris of the battlefield.

IV. Abatement. The absorption and elimination of exudates, pus, etc., take place during the period of abatement. It is accompanied by a gradual lowering of temperature, pulse rate and the other symptoms of fever and inflammation.

V. Resolution or Reconstruction. When the period of Abate-ment has run its course and the affected areas have been cleared of the morbid accumulations and obstructions, then, during the fifth stage of inflammation, the work of rebuilding the injured parts and organs begins. More or less destruction has taken place in the cells and tissues, the blood vessels and organs of the areas involved. These must now be reconstructed, and this last stage of the inflammatory process is, therefore, in a way the most important. On the perfect regeneration of the injured parts depends the final effect of the acute disease upon the organism.

If the inflammation has been allowed to run its course through the different stages of acute activity and the final stage of Reconstruction, then every acute disease, whatever its name and description may be, will prove beneficial to the organism because morbid matter, foreign bodies, poisons and microorganisms have been eliminated from the system; abnormal and diseased tissues have been broken down and built up again to a purer and more normal condition.

As it were, the acute disease has acted upon the organism like a thunderstorm on the sultry, vitiated summer air. It has cleared the system of impurities and destructive influences, and re-established wholesome, normal conditions. Therefore acute diseases, when treated in harmony with Nature's intent, always prove beneficial.

If, however, through neglect or wrong treatment, the inflammatory processes are not allowed to run their natural course, if they are checked or suppressed by poisonous drugs, the ice bag or surgical operations, or if the disease conditions in the system are so far in the ascendancy that the healing forces cannot react properly, then the constructive forces may lose the battle and the disease may take a fatal ending or develop into chronic ailments.

Suppression During the First

Two Stages of Inflammation

It may be suggested that suppression during the stages of Incubation and Aggravation need not have fatal consequences if followed by natural living and eliminative treatment. To this I would reply: "Such procedure always involves the danger of concentrating the disease poisons in vital parts and organs, thus laying the foundation for chronic destructive diseases."

Furthermore, it is not at all necessary to suppress inflammatory processes by poisonous drugs and other unnatural means, because we can easily and surely control them and keep them from becoming dangerous by our natural means of treatment.

I shall now endeavor to prove and to illustrate the foregoing theoretical expositions by following the development of various diseases through the five stages of inflammation. I shall first take up the commonest of all forms of disease, the cold.

Catching a Cold

According to popular opinion, the catching of colds is responsible for the greater portion of human ailments. Almost daily I hear from patients who come for consultation: All my troubles date back to a cold I took at such and such a time, etc. Then I have to explain that colds are not taken suddenly and from without but that they come from within, that their period of Incubation may have extended over months or years, that a clean, healthy body possessed of good vitality cannot take cold under the ordinary thermal conditions congenial to human life, no matter how sudden the change in temperature.

At first glance, this may seem to be contrary to common experience as well as to the theory and practice of medical science. But let us follow the development of a cold from start to finish. This will throw some light on the question as to whether it can be caught, or whether it develops slowly within the organism; also whether this development or incubation may extend over a long period of time.

Taking cold may be caused by chilling of the surface of the body or part of the body. In the chilled portions of the skin the pores close, the blood recedes into the interior, and as a result of this the elimination of poisonous gases and exudates through these portions of the skin is suppressed.

This catching a cold through being exposed to a cold draft, through wet clothing, etc., is not necessarily followed by more serious consequences. If the system is not too much encumbered with morbid matter and if kidneys and intestines are in fairly good working order, these organs will take care of the extra amount of waste and morbid materials in place of the temporarily inactive skin and eliminate them without difficulty. The greater the vitality and the more normal the composition of the blood, the better the system will react in such an emergency and throw off the morbid matter which failed to be eliminated through the skin.

If, however, the organism is already overloaded with waste and morbid materials, if the bowels and the kidneys are already weakened and atrophied through continued overwork and overstimulation, if, in addition to this, the vitality has been lowered through excesses or overexertion and the vital fluids are in an abnormal condition, then the morbid matter thrown into the circulation by the chilling and temporary inactivity of the skin cannot find an outlet through the regular channels of elimination and endeavors to escape by way of the mucous linings of the nasal passages, the throat, bronchi, stomach, bowels and genitourinary organs.

The waste materials and poisonous exudates which are being eliminated through these internal membranes cause irritation and congestion, and thus produce the well-known symptoms of inflammation and catarrhal elimination: sneezing (coryza), cough, expectoration, mucous discharges, diarrhea, leucorrhea [vaginal dis-charge], etc. In other words, these so-called colds are nothing more or less than different forms of vicarious elimination. The membranous linings of the internal organs are doing the work for the inactive, sluggish and atrophied skin, kidneys and intestines. The greater the accumulation of morbid matter in the system, the lower the vitality, and the more abnormal the composition of the blood and lymph, the greater will be the liability to the catching of colds.

What is to be gained by suppressing the different forms of catarrhal elimination with cough and catarrh cures containing opiates, astringents, antiseptics, germkillers and antipyretics? Is it not obvious that such a procedure interferes with Nature's purifying efforts, that it hinders and suppresses the inflammatory processes and the accompanying elimination of morbid matter from the system? Worst of all, that it adds drug poisons to disease poisons?

Such a course can have but one result, namely the changing of Nature's cleansing and healing efforts into chronic disease.

From the foregoing it will have become clear that the cause of a cold lies not so much in the cold draft, or the wet feet, as in the primary causes of all disease: lowered vitality, deterioration of the vital fluids and the accumulation of morbid matter and poisons in the system.

The incubation period of the cold may have extended over many years or over an entire lifetime.

What, then, is the natural cure for colds? There can be but one remedy: increased elimination through the proper channels. This is accomplished by judicious dieting and fasting, and through restoring the natural activity of the skin, kidneys and bowels by means of wet packs, cold sprays and ablutions, sitz baths, massage, chiropractic or osteopathic manipulation, homeopathic remedies, exercise, sun and air baths and all other methods of natural treatment that save vitality, build up the blood on a normal basis and promote elimination without injuring the organism.

Suppression During the Third

Stage of Inflammation

Should the inflammatory processes be suppressed during the stage of Destruction, the results would be still more serious and far-reaching. We have learned that during this stage the affected parts and organs are involved in more or less disintegration. They are filled with morbid exudates, pus, etc., which interfere with and make impossible normal nutrition and functioning. If suppression takes place during this stage, it is obvious that the affected areas will be left permanently in a condition of destruction.

Here is an illustration from practical life: Suppose necessary changes and repairs have to be made in a house. Workmen have torn down the partitions, hangings, wallpaper, etc. At this stage of the proceedings the owner discharges the workmen and the house is left in a condition of chaos. Surely, this would not be rational. It would leave the house unfit for habitation. But such a procedure would correspond exactly to the suppression of inflammatory diseases during the stage of Destruction. This also leaves the affected organs permanently in an abnormal, diseased condition.

That accounts for the mysterious sequelae or chronic after-effects which so often follow drug-treated acute diseases. I have traced numerous cases of chronic affections of the lungs and kidneys, of infantile paralysis and of many other chronic ailments to such suppression. In the following I shall describe a typical case, which came under our care and treatment a few years ago.

Suppression by Means of the Ice Bag

A few years ago several gentlemen of Greek nationality called on me with the request that I visit a friend of theirs who had been lying sick for about two months in one of our great West Side [Chicago] hospitals. On investigation I found that the patient had entered the hospital suffering from a mild case of pneumonia. The doctors of the institution had ordered ice packs. Rubber sheets filled with ice were applied to the chest and other parts of the body. This had been done for several weeks until the fever subsided.

As a matter of fact, ice is more suppressive than antifever medicines. The continued icy cold applications chill the parts of the body to which they are applied, depress the vital functions and effectually suppress the inflammatory processes.

The result in this case, as in many similar ones which I had occasion to observe during and after the ice-bag treatment, was that the inflammation in the lungs had been arrested and suppressed during the stage of destruction, when the air cells and tissues were filled with exudates, blood serum, pus, live and dead blood cells, bacteria, etc., leaving the affected areas of the lungs in a consolidated, liver-like condition.

As a consequence of suppression in the case of this Greek patient, the pneumonia had been changed from the acute to the subacute and chronic stages and the doctors in charge had told his friends that he was now suffering from miliary tuberculosis, and would probably die within a week or two.

After receiving this discouraging information, the friends of the patient came to me and prevailed upon me to take charge of the case. He was transferred to our institution, and we began at once to apply the natural methods of treatment. Instead of ice packs we used the regular cold-water packs, strips of linen wrung out of water of ordinary temperature wrapped around the body and covered with several layers of flannel bandages.

The wet packs became warm on the body in a few minutes. They relaxed the pores and drew the blood into the surface, thus promoting heat radiation and the elimination of morbid matter through the skin. They did not suppress the fever, but kept it below the danger point.

Under this treatment, accompanied by fasting and judicious osteopathic manipulation, the inflammatory and feverish processes suppressed by the ice packs soon revived, became once more active and aggressive, and were now allowed to run their natural course through the stages of destruction, absorption (abatement) and reconstruction.

The result of the Nature Cure treatment was that about two months after the patient entered our institution, his friends bought him a ticket to sunny Greece. He had a good journey, and in the congenial climate of his native country made a perfect recovery.

I have observed a number of similar cases suffering from consolidation of the lungs and the resulting asthmatic or tubercular conditions, which had been doctored into these chronic ailments by means of antipyretics and of ice.

Equally dangerous is the ice bag if applied to the inflamed brain or the spinal column. Only too often it results either in paralysis or in death. In many instances, acute cerebrospinal meningitis is changed in this way by drug and serum treatment or by the use of ice bags into the chronic, so-called incurable infantile paralysis.

We say so-called incurable because we have treated and cured such cases in all stages of development from the acute inflammatory meningitis to the chronic paralysis of long standing.

In our treatment of acute diseases we never use ice or icy water for packs, compresses, baths or ablutions, but always water of ordinary temperature as it comes from the faucet. The water compress or pack warms up quickly, and thus brings about a natural reaction within a few minutes, while the ice bag or pack continually chills and practically freezes the affected parts and organs. This does not allow the skin to relax; it prevents a warm reaction, the radiation of the body heat and the elimination of morbid matter through the skin.

Suppression During the Fourth and Fifth Stages of Inflammation

Let us see what happens when acute diseases are suppressed during the stages of abatement and reconstruction. If the defenders of the body, the phagocyte and antitoxins, produced in the tissues and organs, gain the victory over the inimical forces which are threatening the health and life of the organism, then the symptoms of inflammation, swelling, redness, heat, pain and the accelerated heart action which accompanies them, gradually subside. The debris of the battlefield is carried away through the venous circulation which forms the drainage system of the body.

When in this way all morbid materials have been completely eliminated, Vital Force, "the physician within," will commence to regenerate and reconstruct the injured and destroyed cells and tissues.

If, however, these processes of elimination and reconstruction are interfered with or interrupted before they are completed, then the affected parts and organs will not have a chance to become entirely well or strong. They will remain in an abnormal, crippled condition, and their functional activity will be seriously handicapped.

The After-effects of Drug-Treated Typhoid Fever

In hundreds of cases I have told patients after a glance into their eyes that they were suffering from chronic indigestion, malassimi-lation and malnutrition caused by drug-treated typhoid fever; and every time the records in the eyes were confirmed by the history of the patient.

In such cases the outer rim of the iris shows a wreath of whitish or drug-colored circular flakes. I have named this wreath "the typhoid rosary." It corresponds to the lymphatic and other absorbent vessels in the intestines, and appears in the iris of the eye when these structures have been injured or atrophied by drug, ice or surgical treatment. Wherever this has been done, the venous and lymphatic vessels in the intestines do not absorb the food materials and these pass through the digestive tract and out of the body without being properly digested and assimilated.

During the destructive stages of typhoid fever, the intestines become denuded by the sloughing of their membranous linings. These sloughed membranes give the stools of the typhoid fever patient their peculiar pea soup appearance. In a similar manner the lymphatic, venous and glandular structures which constitute the absorbent vessels of the intestines atrophy and slough away.

If the inflammatory processes are allowed to run their normal course under natural methods of treatment through the stages of Destruction, Absorption and Reconstruction, Nature will rebuild the membranous and glandular structures of the intestinal canal perfectly, convalescence will be rapid and the patient will enjoy better health than before he contracted the disease.

If, however, through injudicious feeding or the administration of quinine, mercury, purging salts, opiates or other destructive agents, Nature's processes are interfered with, prematurely checked and suppressed, then the sloughed membranes and absorbent vessels are not reconstructed, and the intestinal tract is left in a denuded and atrophied condition.

Such a patient may arise from his bed thinking that he is cured; but unless he is afterward treated by natural methods, he will never make a full recovery. It will take him, perhaps, months or years to die a gradual, miserable death through malassimilation and malnutrition, which usually end in some form of wasting disease, such as pernicious anemia or tuberculosis. If he does not actually die from the effects of the wrongly treated typhoid fever, he will be troubled all his life with intestinal indigestion, constipation, malassimilation and the accompanying nervous disorders.

A Change for the Better

Speaking of typhoid fever, we are glad to say that for this particular form of disease the most advanced medical science has adopted the Nature Cure treatment, that is, straight cold water and fasting, and no drugs, as it was originated by the pioneers of Nature Cure in Germany more than fifty years ago.

This treatment, which medical science has found so eminently successful in typhoid fever, would prove equally efficacious in all other acute diseases if the regular doctors would only try it. It is a strange and curious fact that so far they have never found it worth while to do so. All Nature Cure physicians know from their daily experience in actual practice that the simple water treatment and fasting is sufficient to cure all other forms of acute diseases just as easily and effectively as typhoid fever. By this is proved the unity of treatment in all acute diseases.

Both in typhoid fever and in tuberculosis, progressive medical men have now entirely abandoned the germ-killing method of treatment. They have found it absolutely useless and superfluous to hunt for drugs and serums to kill the typhoid and tuberculosis bacilli in these, the two most destructive diseases afflicting the human family. They were forced to admit that the simple remedies of the Nature Cure school, cold water and fasting in typhoid fever and the fresh-air treatment in tuberculosis, are the only worthwhile methods to fight these formidable enemies to health and life.

If they would continue their researches and experiments along these natural lines, they would attain infinitely more satisfactory results than through their germ-hunting and germ-killing theories and practices.

Chapter IX

The Effects of Suppression of Venereal Diseases

Another good illustration of suppression may be found in the allopathic treatment of venereal diseases. Almost invariably the drug treatment suppresses these diseases in the stages of incubation and aggravation, thus locking them up in the system. The venereal taints and germs, however, are living things which grow and multiply until the body has been completely permeated by them. Then they must find an outlet somehow and somewhere, and consequently they break out in the manifold so-called "secondary" and "tertiary" symptoms.

The drug poisons which are used to "cure" (suppress) these symptoms, greatly aggravate the disease. They create conditions in the system infinitely worse than the venereal diseases themselves. Thus the acute, easily curable stages of these ailments are changed into the dreadful and obstinate chronic conditions. It is in this way that venereal diseases are made hereditary and transmitted to future generations.

In a special article on this subject entitled "Venereal Diseases," published in ~"The Naturopath,"~ January, 1913, I have substantiated the following claims:

"Venereal diseases are not necessarily chronic in their progressive development. "They are essentially acute and self-limited. But may become chronic through neglect or through suppressive drug treatment. "The chronic, so-called secondary and tertiary manifestations of venereal diseases, such as ulceration of bones and fleshy tissue, gummata of the brain, sclerosis of the spinal cord, arthritic rheumatism, degeneration and destruction of other vital parts and organs of the body, are not so much the result of the original gonorrheal or syphilitic infection, as of the destructive drug poisons which have been taken to cure or rather to suppress the primary lesions and acute inflammatory symptoms. "Venereal diseases in the acute inflammatory stages are easily and completely curable by natural methods of living and of treatment. "Venereal diseases treated and cured by natural methods during the acute inflammatory stages are never followed by any chronic after-effects or secondary and tertiary manifestations whatsoever. "When venereal diseases have reached the secondary and tertiary stages, they are still curable by natural methods of living and of treatment, providing there is left sufficient vitality to respond to treatment and providing the destruction of vital parts and organs has not advanced too far.

"Hundreds of cases of well-developed locomotor ataxy, paresis, and other so-called secondary and tertiary diseases of the brain and the nervous system, of bony and fleshy tissues, and of vital organs have been cured by our natural methods of treatment.

"It is self-evident, however, that the treatment and cure of the chronic conditions require more patience and perseverance than the cure of acute conditions not tampered with and suppressed by drugs. "Venereal diseases treated and cured by natural methods are never followed by chronic after-effects. On the other hand, mercury, iodine, quinine, and coal-tar poisons produce all the so-called secondary and tertiary symptoms of syphilis in people who never in their lives were afflicted with venereal diseases, but who have taken or absorbed these drug poisons in other ways.

". . . These facts are proven beyond doubt by the Diagnosis from the Eye. All, destructive poisons taken in sufficient quantities will in time reveal their presence and exact location in the body through certain well-defined signs or discolorations in the iris.

"These poisons undermine the structures of the body and deteriorate vital parts and organs so slowly and insidiously that the superficial observer does not trace and connect cause and effect."

The Wasserman and Noguchi Tests

Medical men may say to the foregoing that the Wasserman and Noguchi tests furnish positive proofs of syphilis in the system. These chemical tests are supposed to reveal with certainty the presence of venereal taints in the body,—at least, the public is left under this impression.

I am convinced, however, that in many instances the "positive" Wasserman or Noguchi tests are the result of mercurial poison instead of syphilitic infection. In a number of cases where these tests proved "positive," that is, where, according to the theory of allopathic medical science, they indicated a luetic condition of the system, the subjects of these tests had never in their lives shown any symptoms of syphilis nor, as far as they knew, had they ever been exposed to infection, but every one of them showed plainly the sign of mercurial poisoning in the iris of the eye, and had taken considerable mercury in the form of calomel or of other medicinal preparations for diseases not of a luetic nature, or they had been "salivated" by coming in contact with the mercurial poison in mines, smelters, mirror factories, etc.

This leads me to believe that, sooner or later, medical science will have to admit that the Wasserman and Noguchi tests reveal, in many instances at least, the effects of mercurial poisoning instead of the effects of syphilitic infection. And this would not be surprising since it is well known that mercury has very similar effects upon the system as syphilis.

It takes the mercurial poison from five to ten and even fifteen years before it works its way into the brain and spinal cord, and there causes its characteristic degeneration and destruction of brain and nerve tissues which manifest outwardly as locomotor ataxy, paralysis agitans, paresis, apoplexy, hemiplegia, epilepsy, St. Vitus dance, and the different forms of idiocy and insanity. Mercurial poisoning is also in many instances the cause of deafness and blindness.

When the symptoms of mercurial destruction begin to show, then they, in turn, are suppressed by preparations of iodine, the "606," or other "alteratives," and so the merry war goes, on: poison against poison, Beelzebub against the Devil, and the poor suffering body has to stand it all.

In this way the system is periodically saturated with the most virulent poisons on earth, until the undertaker finishes the job. And this is miscalled "scientific treatment." There never was invented by cruel Indian or fanatical inquisition worse torture than this. They mercifully finished the sufferings of their victims within a few hours or, at the worst, days; but this torture inflicted upon human beings in the name of medical science continues for a lifetime. It means dying by inches under the most horrible conditions for ten, twenty, thirty years or longer.

In this connection it may be well to quote the testimony of Professor E. A. Farrington of Philadelphia, one of the most celebrated homeopathic physicians of the nineteenth century. He says, in his ~"Clinical Materia Medica,"~ third edition, page 141:

"The various constitutions or dyscrasia underlying chronic and acute affections are, indeed, very numerous. As yet, we do not know them all. We do know that one of them comes in gonorrhoea, a disease which is frightfully common, so that the constitution arising from this disease is rapidly on the increase.

"Now I want to tell you why it is so. It is because allopathic physicians, and many homeopaths as well, do not properly cure it. I do not believe gonorrhoea to be a local disease. If it is not properly cured, a constitutional poison which may be transmitted to the children is developed. I know, from years of experience and observation, that gonorrhoea is a serious difficulty, and one, too, that complicates many cases that we have to treat.

"The same is true of syphilis in a modified degree. Gonorrhoea seems to attack the nobler tissues, the lungs, the heart, and the nervous system, all of which are reached by syphilis only after the lapse of years."

The Destructive After-Effects of Mercury

Concerning the destructive after-effects of mercury, of which homeopaths have made a most careful study, Professor Farrington says, on pages 558-559 of the same volume:

"The more remote symptoms of mercurial poisoning are these: You will find that the blood becomes impoverished. The albumin and fibrin of that fluid are affected. They are diminished, and you find in their place a certain fatty substance, the composition of which I do not exactly know. Consequently, as a prominent symptom, the body wastes and emaciates. The patient suffers from fever which is rather hectic in its character. The periosteum becomes affected, and you then have a characteristic group of mercurial pains, bone pains worse in changes of the weather, worse in the warmth of the bed, and chilliness with or after stool. The skin becomes rather of a brownish hue; ulcers form, particularly on the legs; they are stubborn and will not heal. The patient is troubled with sleeplessness and ebullitions of blood at night; he is hot and cannot sleep; he is thrown quickly into a perspiration, which perspiration gives him no relief.

"The entire system suffers also, and you have here two series of symptoms. At first the patient becomes anxious and restless and cannot remain quiet; he changes his position; he moves about from place to place; he seems to have a great deal of anxiety about the heart, praecordial anguish, as it is termed, particularly at night.

"Then, in another series of symptoms, there are jerkings of the limbs, making the patient appear as though he were attacked by St. Vitus' dance. Or, you may notice what is more common yet, trembling of the hands, this tremor being altogether beyond the control of the patient and gradually spreading over the entire body, giving you a resemblance to paralysis agitans or shaking palsy.

"Finally, the patient becomes paralyzed, cannot move his limbs, his mind becomes lost, and he presents a perfect picture of imbecility. He does all sorts of queer things. He sits in the corner with an idiotic smile on his face, playing with straws; he is forgetful, he cannot remember even the most ordinary events. He becomes disgustingly filthy and eats his own excrement. In fact, he is a perfect idiot.

"Be careful how you give mercury; it is a treacherous medicine. It seems often indicated. You give it and relieve; but your patient is worse again in a few weeks and then you give it again with relief. By and by, it fails you. Now, if I want to make a permanent cure, for instance, in a scrofulous child, I will very seldom give him mercury; should I do so, it will be at least only as an intercurrent remedy."

Chapter X

Suppressive Surgical Treatment of Tonsillitis and Enlarged Adenoids

The following paragraphs are taken from an article in the ~Nature Cure Magazine~ May, 1909, titled "Surgery for Tonsillitis and Adenoids." They will throw further interesting light on the dangerous consequences of suppressing acute and subacute diseases.

"The tonsils are excreting glands. Nature has created them for the elimination of impurities from the body. Acute, subacute and chronic tonsillitis accompanied by enlargement and cheesy decay of the tonsils means that these glands have been habitually congested with morbid matter and poisons, that they have had more work to do than they could properly attend to.

"These glandular structures constitute a valuable part of the drainage system of the organism. If the blood is poisoned through overeating and faulty food combinations, or with scrofulous, venereal or psoriatic poisons, the tonsils are called upon, along with other organs, to eliminate these morbid taints. Is it any wonder that frequently they become inflamed and subject to decay? What, however, can be gained by destroying them with iodine or extirpating them with the surgeon's scissors or the 'guillotine'?

"Because your servants are weakened by overwork, would you kill them? Because the drains in your house are too small to carry off the waste, would you blockade or remove them? Still, this is the orthodox philosophy of the medical schools applied to the management of the human body.

". . . In case of any morbid discharge from the body, wherever it be, whether through hemorrhoids, open sores, ulcers or through tonsils, scrofulous glands, etc., a fontanelle has been established to which and through which systemic poisons make their way. If such an outlet be blocked by medical or surgical treatment the stream of morbid matter has to seek another escape or else the poisons will accumulate somewhere in the body.

"Fortunate is the patient when such an escape can be established, because wherever in the system morbid excretions, suppressed by medical treatment, concentrate, there will inevitably be found the seat of chronic disease.

"After the tonsils have been removed, the morbid matter which they were eliminating usually finds the nearest and easiest outlet through the adenoid tissues and nasal membranes. These now take up the work of 'vicarious' elimination and, in their turn, become hyperactive and inflamed.

"Sometimes it happens that the adenoid tissues become affected before the tonsils. In that case, also, relief through the surgeon's knife is sought and then the process is reversed: after the adenoids have been removed, the tonsils develop chronic catarrhal conditions.

"When both tonsils and adenoids have been removed, the nasal membranes will, in turn, become congested and swollen. Often the mucous elimination increases to an alarming degree, and frequently polyps and other growths make their appearance or the turbinated bones soften and swell and obstruct the nasal passages, thus again making the patient a 'mouth breather.'

"But in vain does Nature protest against local symptomatic treatment. Science has nothing to learn from her.

"When the nose takes up the work of vicarious elimination, the same mode of treatment is resorted to. The mucous membranes of the nose are now swabbed and sprayed with antiseptics and astringents, or 'burned' by cauterizers, electricity, etc. The polyps are cut out, and frequently parts of the turbinated bone and septum as well, in order to open the air passages.

"Now, surely, the patient must be cured. But, strange to say, new and more serious troubles arise. The posterior nasal passages and the throat are now affected by chronic catarrhal conditions and there is much annoyance from phlegm and mucous discharges which drop into the throat. These catarrhal conditions frequently extend to the mucous membranes of stomach and intestines.

"When the drainage system of the nose and the nasopharyngeal cavities has been completely destroyed, the impurities must either travel upward into the brain or downward into the glandular structures of the neck, thence into the bronchi and the tissues of the lungs.

"If the trend be upward, to the brain, the patient grows nervous and irritable or becomes dull and apathetic. How often is a child reprimanded or even punished for laziness and inattention when it cannot help itself? In many instances the morbid matter affects certain centers in the brain and causes nervous conditions, hysteria, St. Vitus' dance, epilepsy, etc. In children the impurities frequently find an outlet through the eardrums in the form of pus-like discharges. This may frequently avert inflammation of the brain, meningitis, imbecility, insanity or infantile paralysis.

"If the trend of the suppressed impurities and poisons be downward, it often results in the hypertrophy and degeneration of the lymphatic glands of the neck. In such cases the suppressive treatment, by drugs or knife, is again applied instead of eliminative and curative measures. The scrofulous poisons, suppressed and driven back from the diseased glands in the neck, now find lodgment in the bronchi and lungs, where they accumulate and form a luxuriant soil for the growth of the bacilli of pneumonia and tuberculosis.

"In other cases, the vocal organs become seriously affected by chronic catarrhal conditions, abnormal growths and in later stages by tuberculosis. Many a fine voice has been ruined in this way.

"The prevention and the cure of all these ailments lie not in local symptomatic treatment and suppression by drugs or knife, but in the rational and natural treatment of the body as a whole."

Chapter XI

Cancer

Let us see how our theories of the Unity of Disease and Cure apply to cancer, the much-dreaded and rapidly increasing disease which is considered absolutely incurable by both the laity and the medical profession.

Allopathy says that the only possible remedy is "early operation." Nevertheless, in the textbooks of medical science and in medical schools and colleges it is taught that cancer and all other malignant growths "always return after extirpation." In fact, every student of medicine is expected to state this in his examination papers as part of the definition of malignant tumors.

The great majority of medical practitioners hold, furthermore, that cancer is a local disease. This is proved by the fact that they apply local, symptomatic treatment.

In reality, however, the disease is constitutional. Therefore, after removal of the growth by surgery, the electric needle, x-rays, etc., the cancer or tumor is liable to break out again in the same place or in several places.

The surest way to change insignificant, so-called "benign" (not fatal to life) fibroid or fatty tumors into malignant cancer or sarcoma is to operate upon them. Wens and warts are often made malignant by surgical interference or other local irritation.

In my article titled "What We Know About Cancer" in the August, 1909, issue of the ~Nature Cure Magazine~ I quote from an article by Burton J. Hendrick, the cancer expert, published in the July, 1909, number of ~McClure's Magazine,~ as follows:

"Clinical observation long ago established the fact that any irritating interference with a cancer almost always stimulates its growth. In his earliest experiments Dr. Loeb found that, by merely drawing a silk thread through a dormant or slowly developing tumor, he could transform it into a rapidly growing one. Cutting with a knife produced the same effect. This accounts for the commonly observed fact that, when extirpated cancers in human beings recur, they increase in size much more rapidly than the original growth."

The late Dr. Senn, the great cancer surgeon, admitted these facts in an interview given to Chicago press representatives upon his return from his trip around the world in 1906. The press clipping reads as follows.

"Avoid Beauty Doctors"

"Incidentally, Dr. Senn advises women who worry over their disfigurement of moles about their heads and shoulders to have those so-called beauty spots removed early in life, but he tells them they should not go to beauty doctors to have the operations performed.

"He knows of hundreds of cases, he says, where cancer has resulted from the irritation of moles by an electric needle, or by constant picking it. 'Have a surgeon cut the mole out,' is his advice, as it will hurt little and leave no scar."

To this we answered in our comments on the interview: "If the little knife of the beauty doctor causes cancer, what about the big knife of the surgeon?"

In point of fact, our office records show that a large percentage of malignant growths are the direct result of surgical operations.

Cancer Not a Local, But a Constitutional Disease

For many years I have been teaching in my lectures and writings as well as in private advice to patients that cancer is a constitutional disease; that it is rooted in every drop of blood in the body; that it is caused by the presence of certain disease taints or of food and drug poisons in the system; that these poisons irritate and stimulate the cells in a certain locality and cause their abnormal multiplication or proliferation in the forms of benign or malignant tumors.

I also claim that meat eating has much to do with the causation of cancer.

Certain discoveries by Dr. H. C. Ross of London, England, confirm my claims that cancer is not at all of local and accidental origin, but that it is constitutional, and that it may be caused by the gradual accumulation in the system of certain poisons which form in decaying animal matter.

One day, while experimenting in his laboratory, Dr. Ross brought white blood cells or leucocytes into contact with a certain aniline dye on the slide of a microscope and noticed that they began at once to multiply by cell division (proliferation). This was the first time that cell proliferation had been observed by the human eye while the cells were separated from their parent organism.

Dr. Ross realized that he had made an important discovery and continued his experiments under the microscope in order to find out what other substances would cause cell multiplication. He found that certain xanthines and albuminoids derived from decaying animal matter were the most effective for this purpose and induced more rapid cell proliferation than any other substances he was able to procure.

Dr. Ross obtained these "alkaloids of putrefaction," as he called them, from blood which had been allowed to putrefy in a warm place. He found that albuminoids derived from decaying vegetable substances did not have the same effect.

His discoveries led him to believe that the alkaloids of putrefaction produced in a cut or wound by the decaying of dead blood and tissue cells are the cause of the rapid multiplication of the neighboring live cells, which gradually fill the wound with new tissues.

Thus, for the first time in the history of medicine, a rational explanation of Nature's methods for repairing injured tissues has been advanced.

Dr. Ross applied his theory still farther to the causation of benign and malignant growths, reasoning that the alkaloids of putrefaction produced in or attracted to a certain part of the body by some local irritation are the cause of the rapid, abnormal multiplication of cells in tumor formations.

In benign tumors the abnormal proliferation of cells takes place slowly, and they do not tend to immediate and rapid decay and deterioration.

In malignant tumors the "wild" cells, created in immense numbers, decay almost as rapidly as they are produced because the abnormal growths are devoid of normal organization. They have no established, regular blood and nerve supply, nor are they provided with adequate venous drainage. They are, therefore, cut off from the orderly life of the organism and doomed to rapid deterioration.

The processes of decay of these tumor materials liberate large quantities of alkaloids of putrefaction, and these, in turn, stimulate the normal, healthy cells with which they come in contact to rapid, abnormal multiplication.

The malignant growth, therefore, feeds on its own products of decay, aside from the systemic poisons and morbid materials already contained in the blood and tissues of the body. These morbid products permeate the entire system. They are carried by the circulation of the blood into all parts of the body. This explains why cancer is a constitutional disease, why it is, as I stated it, "rooted in every drop of blood."

It also explains why cancer, or rather the disposition to its development (diathesis), is hereditary.

If the original cancerous growth is removed by surgical intervention, x-rays, the electric needle, cauterization or any other form of local treatment, the poisonous materials (alkaloids of putrefaction) in the blood will set up other foci of abnormal, wild proliferation. Medical science has applied the term metastasis to such spreading and reappearing of malignant tumors after extirpation.

Dr. Ross' findings throw an interesting light on the relationship between cancer and meat eating. Is it not self-evident that in a digestive tract filled most of the time with large masses of partially digested and decaying animal food enormous quantities of alkaloids of putrefaction are created? These are absorbed into the circulation, attracted to any point where exists some form of local irritation and then stimulate the cells in that locality to abnormal proliferation.

"But," it will be said, "meat eating alone does not account for cancer, because vegetarians also succumb to the disease." This is true. Alkaloids of putrefaction are constantly produced in every animal and human body. They form in the excretions of living cells and in the decaying protoplasm of dead cells, and if the organs of elimination do not function properly, these morbid materials will accumulate in the system.

Furthermore, the Diagnosis from the Eye furnishes positive proof that Hahnemann's theory of psora is based on truth. I quote from my article in the ~Nature Cure Magazine~ August, 1909:

"For a hundred years, Hahnemann's theory of psora has been scouted and ridiculed by the allopathic schools and even among homeopaths only a few have accepted it. Now we are confronted by the remarkable fact that, at this late day, the Diagnosis from the Eye confirms the observations and speculations of the great genius of homeopathy.

"After suppression of itchy eruptions, lice, crab lice, etc., spots ranging in color from light brown to dark red appear in different places in the iris of the eye. These 'itch spots' indicate the organs and localities of the body in which the suppressed disease taints have concentrated.

"Such suppressions represent not only the scrofulous taints which Nature was trying to eliminate by means of eruptions and parasites, but, in addition to these, the poisons contained in the bodies of the parasites and the drug poisons which were used to suppress or kill them.

"It has been found that the bodies of the itch parasites (~Sarcoptes scabici~) contain an exceedingly poisonous substance which the homeopaths call 'psorinum'. When these minute animals burrowing in and under the skin are killed by poisonous drugs and antiseptics, the morbid taints in their bodies are absorbed by the system and added to the psoriatic poisons which Nature has been trying to eliminate.

"Thus, after suppression of itchy eruptions or parasites, the organism is encumbered with three poisons instead of one: (1) the hereditary or acquired scrofulous and psoriatic taints which the cells of the body were throwing off into the blood stream and which the blood was feeding to the parasites on the surface, (2) the morbid substance contained in the bodies of the parasites, (3) the drug poisons used as suppressants. (Such poisons may lie latent in the system for many years before they become active and, in combination with other disease taints and with food and drug poisons, create the different forms of chronic destructive diseases.)

"These facts explain why the itch spots in different areas of the iris of the eye so frequently indicate serious chronic, destructive disease conditions in the parts and organs of the body corresponding to these areas, why; for instance, in asthma and tuberculosis we often find itch spots in the region representing the lungs or why in cancer of the liver or of the stomach itch spots show in the area of stomach or liver.

"That the itch or psoriatic taint is actually at the bottom of the cancerous diathesis is attested by the fact that all cancer patients whom we have treated and cured, with two exceptions (whose healing crisis took the form of furunculosis), broke out with the itch at one time or another during the natural treatment. In most of these cases the bodies of the patients were inflamed with fiery eruptions for days or even weeks at a time.

"Nature Cure allows these healing crises to run their course unhindered and unchecked; in fact, we encourage them by air and sun baths, cold-water treatment and homeopathic remedies."

What has been said verifies my claim that benign and malignant tumors can be cured only by thorough purifying the system of all morbid and poisonous taints and by building up the blood to a normal basis, that is, by providing it with the proper elements of nutrition, especially with the all-important organic salts.

That this is not merely theory, but actual fact has been proved in the great cancer institutes in Europe and in this country. The scientists in charge of these institutions report that they have found a positive cure for cancer in animals. The treatment is as follows:

The blood is pumped out of the body of a dog or other animal afflicted with cancer and immediately afterwards the blood of a healthy animal which has shown immunity to cancer inoculation is pumped into the body of the diseased animal. It is reported that in nine cases out of ten thus treated the cancerous growths disappear.

This treatment, of course, entails the death of the animal which had to give up its life blood to cure the other and therefore this method of cure is not adaptable to human beings. Even though an individual, with suicidal intent, would be willing to give up his life for a stipulated legacy to his relatives, the law would not sanction the transaction.

However, we of the Nature Cure school say that it is not necessary to pump the diseased blood out of the organism. In the natural methods of living and of treatment we possess the means of purifying and regenerating that blood while it is in the body. That this is possible we have proved in a number of cancer cases.

It is obvious, however, that the earlier the disease is treated by the natural methods, that is, before the breaking-down process has far advanced, the easier and quicker will be the cure.

In the case of tumors, then, we see again verified the fundamental law of Nature Cure: the Unity of Disease and of Treatment. We see that the tumor is not of local, but of constitutional, origin, that its period of incubation may extend over a lifetime or over several generations.

Chapter XII

Women's Suffering

Certain ailments peculiar to the female organism have become almost universal among civilized races. Probably the majority of surgical operations are performed for so-called women's diseases. That women suffer untold agonies during menstruation, in childbirth and at the climacteric is looked upon as unavoidable and a matter of course.

The fact that the native women of Africa, of the Sandwich Islands, the South American bush and our western plains are practically exempt from these ailments indicates that the cause of female troubles must lie in artificial habits of living and in the unnatural treatment of diseases.

Many are beginning to recognize these truths. For them is dawning a new era, when knowledge will free Woman from physical suffering as it has freed her from other bondage.

Instances like the following are of common occurrence in our free clinics for Diagnosis from the Eye:

A lady tells us that she has been suffering for many years from a complication of female troubles. Her eyes show a heavy scurf rim, indicating an inactive, atrophied skin, poor surface circulation and, as a result of this condition, defective elimination through the skin and accumulation of waste matter and systemic poisons in the system. The areas of stomach and intestines reveal the signs of chronic catarrhal affection and atrophy of the membranous linings and glandular structures. This, of course, means indigestion, fermentation of foods, gas formation, constipation and a multitude of resulting disturbances.

The signs in the iris also indicate an atonic, relaxed and prolapsed condition of stomach, bowels and other abdominal organs. This is likely to cause sagging of the genital organs, relaxation of the bands and ligaments which hold them in place and, as a result of this relaxation, misplacement of the womb.

We tell the patient of our findings in her eyes and she admits all the conditions and symptoms which we describe, but she is not satisfied because our diagnosis does not agree with that of the great specialists and professors of medicine whom she has consulted. Every one of them has told her that all her troubles are due to the fact that her uterus is flexed and retroverted, that it presses on the rectum (this being the cause of her chronic constipation and of the obstructed menstrual flow, the congestion, pain, etc.), and that the womb must be placed in its normal position by a surgical operation.

In this and many similar cases that have come to us for treatment, it was the relaxed and prolapsed condition of the stomach and intestines that caused the sinking (prolapsus) of the uterus with the attending distressing symptoms. In some instances the womb and with it the bladder had fallen so low that they protruded from the vagina. In all of these cases, as the patients without exception told us, the professors and specialists assured them that surgical treatment, shortening of the ligaments, the insertion of pessaries, the cutting loose and raising of the womb, etc., were the only possible means of curing these ailments.

So we explain to the lady that the relaxed and prolapsed condition of the genital organs, the misplacement of the womb, etc., are not causes of disease, but only the effects of the weakened and relaxed condition of the digestive organs, and that this, in turn, is due to indigestion, malnutrition, defective elimination through skin, bowels and kidneys; that, therefore, the only possibility of cure lies in correcting and overcoming these constitutional conditions through an eliminative diet, blood-building remedies and other natural methods; that the blood must be built up on a normal basis, and that the digestive tract and the other abdominal organs must be made more alive and active through hydropathic treatment, massage, spinal manipulation, general and special exercises, air and sun baths, etc.

In thousands of cases we have thus cured female troubles without poisonous drugs or surgical operations, simply by improving the digestion, purifying the blood and invigorating the abdominal organs in a natural manner.

On the other hand, almost daily we meet with instances of untold suffering as the direct consequence of operations, the use of pessaries, etc., which only served to weaken the genital organs still more and resulted in all sorts of complications, inflammations, adhesions, etc., and in many cases in malignant tumors.

In this connection I would warn especially against the use of pessaries. They are at best only a mechanical contrivance, and do not add anything to the improvement of the diseased condition. On the other hand, they irritate the abdominal organs by excessive pressure, which in many instances produces inflammation of the neighboring tissues and abnormal growths.

Suppressing inflammation of the genital organs by poisonous antiseptics, sprays, tampons or other local applications only tends to aggravate the chronic conditions. Curetting (scraping) the womb does not cure the catarrhal affection, but only serves to destroy its delicate mucous lining and to suppress catarrhal elimination. Holding up the womb by means of a pessary in order to strengthen its muscles and ligaments is about as reasonable and effective as to try to strengthen a weak arm by carrying it in a sling. Replacing or removing misplaced or affected organs by means of surgery does not contribute anything toward correcting the causes of these abnormal conditions, but in many instances makes a real cure impossible. How can an organ be cured after it has been extirpated with the knife?

It is a fact known to every observing physician that from fifty to seventy-five percent of all women have some kind of misplacement of the genital organs and that only a comparatively small number of these suffer from local disturbances, indicating that, in most cases, misplacement alone will not create serious trouble.

It is ridiculous to assume that the small, flabby uterus of an anemic woman can block the rectum and cause disease, but it is an excellent talking point, as effective in bringing victims to the operating table as appendicitis with its fairy tales of seeds and foreign bodies lodging in the appendix vermiformis.

While studying Nature Cure in Germany, I took special courses in the Thure-Brandt Massage. By means of this internal manipulative treatment, weakness of ligaments and muscles, displacements, adhesions, etc., can be corrected without the use of knife or drugs. During my first years in practice, I frequently resorted to the internal manual treatment with good results; but I found that in most cases it was not at all necessary in order to produce perfect cures.

I saw that chiropractic and osteopathic correction of spinal and pelvic lesions and consequent removal of irritation and pressure on the nerves, the cure of chronic constipation and malnutrition by pure food diet and hydrotherapy, the strengthening of the pelvic muscles and nerves by means of active and passive movements and exercises, were fully sufficient to correct the local symptoms in a natural manner. Thousands of cases cured by us by these methods attest the truth of our statements; while those who failed to understand the simple reasoning of the Nature Cure philosophy or lacked will power to withstand the arguments of friends and physicians followed the siren call of the operating table and have been sorry for it ever since.

In case of operation for misplacement of the womb, it is necessary, in order to keep the womb in its new position, to stitch it to the frontal abdominal wall. Very frequently it will not stay there, breaks loose, and relapses into an abnormal position. Granted that it remains fixed, woe to the woman if she becomes pregnant. The womb cannot assume the constantly changing positions of pregnancy, and the result is either abortion or malformation of the fetus, together with great and constant suffering to the woman.

The operation has done nothing to correct unnatural habits of living or to purify the system of its scrofulous and psoriatic taints, of drug and food poisons. Frequently these gather in the parts that have been weakened and irritated by the antiseptics and by the surgeon's knife, and set up new inflammations, ulcerations and only too often malignant tumors. As a result, one operation follows another.

We cannot cut in the genital organs without cutting in the brain. The nervous system is a unit, and the brain is directly and intimately connected with the complex and highly sensitive nerve centers of the genital organs. Mutilation of the genital nerve centers, therefore, invariably affects the brain, and thus the intellectual and emotional life of a woman. It is almost axiomatic that a woman whose uterus or ovaries have been removed or mutilated is afterward mentally and emotionally more or less abnormal. Nervousness, irritability and only too often nervous prostration and insanity are the sequelae of operative treatment.

In medical colleges, among students and professors, these facts are freely admitted and discussed, but the prospective patient hears a different story. "Cut loose the womb, shorten the ligaments, put it into the right position, and everything will be well." This sounds plausible and seductive; but everyday experiences expose the inadequacy and the destructive aftereffects of local symptomatic treatment.

The Climacteric or Change of Life

Under our artificial methods of living, the ~climacteric~ or change of life, has become the bugbear of womanhood. It seems to be universally assumed that this period in a woman's life must be fraught with manifold sufferings and dangers. It is taken as a matter of course that during these changes in her organism a woman is assailed by the most serious physical, mental, and psychic ailments which may endanger her sanity and often her life.

Like rheumatism, neurasthenia, neuralgia and hundreds of other medical terms, "change of life" is a convenient phrase to cover the doctor's ignorance. No matter what ailments befall a woman during the years from forty to fifty, may the causes be ever so obscure, the diagnosis is easy. "You are in the climacteric, you are suffering from the change of life," says the doctor, and the patient is satisfied and resigns herself to the inevitable.

Frequently women come to us for consultation, and after reciting a long string of troubles they conclude with the remark: "Of course, doctor, I'm in the change, and I know that lots of these things are natural at my time of life."

Is it true that all this suffering is natural and inevitable? Among the primitive races of the earth suffering incident to the change of life is practically unknown. The same is true in a lesser degree of the country population of Europe. The causes of it must, therefore, be sought in the artificial modes of living peculiar to our hypercivilization and in the unnatural methods of treating disease as commonly practiced.

Which are the specific causes of the profound disturbances so often accompanying the organic changes of the climacteric?

Aside from their other physiological functions, the menses are for the woman a monthly cleansing crisis through which Nature eliminates from her system considerable amounts of waste and morbid matter which, under a natural regime of life, would be discharged by means of the organs of depuration, that is, the lungs, skin, kidneys and bowels.

The more natural the life and the more normal, as the result of this, the woman's physical condition, the shorter and less annoying and painful, within certain limits, will be the menstrual periods.

Through unnatural habits of eating, drinking, dressing, breathing and through equally unnatural methods of medical treatment, the kidneys, skin and bowels have become inactive, benumbed or paralyzed. As long as the vicarious monthly purification by means of the menses continues, the evil results of the torpid condition of the regular organs of depuration do not become so apparent. The organism has learned to adapt itself to this mode of elimination.

But when, on account of the organic changes of the climacteric, menstruation ceases, then the systemic poisons, which formerly were eliminated by means of this monthly purification, accumulate in the system and become the source of all manner of trouble. All tendencies to physical, mental or psychic disease are greatly intensified. The poisonous taints circulating in the blood overstimulate or else depress and paralyze the brain and the nervous system. As a consequence, mental and psychic disorders are of common occurrence; the more so because the waning of the sex

Chapter XIII

The Treatment of Acute Diseases by Natural Methods

In the preceding chapters we have described the results of the wrong, that is, suppressive treatment of acute diseases. We shall now proceed to describe the simple and uniform methods of natural treatment.

If the uniformity of acute diseases be a fact in Nature, then it follows that it must be possible to treat all acute diseases by uniform methods.

That it is possible to treat all acute diseases most successfully by natural methods, which anybody possessed of ordinary intelligence can apply, has been demonstrated for more than seventy years by the Nature Cure practitioners in Germany, and by myself during the last ten years in an extensive practice.

One of the many advantages of natural treatment is that it may be applied right from the beginning, as soon as the first symptoms of acute febrile conditions manifest themselves. It is not necessary to wait for a correct diagnosis of the case.

The regular physician, with his specific treatment for the multitude of specific diseases which he recognizes, often has to wait several days or even weeks before the real nature of the disease becomes clear to him, before he is able to diagnose the case or even to make a good guess. The conscientious medical practitioner has to postpone actual treatment until the symptoms are well defined. Meanwhile he applies expectant treatment as it is called in medical parlance, that is, he gives a purgative or a placebo, something or other to placate, or to make the patient and his friends believe that something is being done.

But during this period of indecision and inaction very often the best opportunity for aiding Nature in her healing efforts is lost, and the inflammatory processes may reach such virulence that it becomes very difficult or even impossible to keep them within constructive limits. The bonfire that was to burn up the rubbish on the premises may, if not watched and tended, assume such proportions that it damages or destroys the house.

It must also be borne in mind that very frequently acute diseases do not present the well-defined sets of symptoms which fit into the accepted medical conception of certain specific ailments. On the contrary, in many instances the symptoms suggest a combination of different forms of acute diseases.

If the character of the disease is ill-defined and complicated, how, then, is the physician of the "Old School" to select the proper specific remedy, Under such circumstances, the diagnosis of the case as well as the medical treatment will at best be largely guesswork.

Compare with this unreliable and unsatisfactory treatment the simple and scientific, exact and efficient natural methods. The natural remedies can be applied from the first, at the slightest manifestation of inflammatory and febrile symptoms. No matter what the specific nature or trend of the inflammatory process, whether it be a simple cold, or whether it take the form of measles, scarlet fever, diphtheria, smallpox, appendicitis, etc.—it makes absolutely no difference in the mode of treatment. In many instances the natural treatment will have broken the virulence of the attack or brought about a cure before the regular physician gets good and ready to apply his specific treatment.

In the following I shall describe briefly these natural methods for the treatment of acute diseases which insure the largest possible percentage of recoveries and at the same time do not in any way tax the system, cause undesirable aftereffects or lead to the different forms of chronic invalidism.

The Natural Remedies

The most important ones of these natural remedies can be had free of cost in any home. They are: air, fasting or eliminative diets, water, and the right mental attitude.

I am fully convinced that these remedies offered freely by Mother Nature are sufficient, if rightly applied, to cure any acute disease arising within the organism. If circumstances permit, however, we may advantageously add corrective manipulation of the spine, massage, magnetic treatment, advanced regenerative modalities (like the Magnatherm) and homeopathic, herbal and specific nutritional supplementation.

The Fresh-Air Treatment

A plentiful supply of pure fresh air is of vital importance at any time. We can live without food for several weeks and without water for several days, but we cannot live without air for more than a few minutes. Just as a fire in the furnace cannot be kept up without a good draft which supplies the necessary amount of oxygen to the flame, so the fires of life in the body cannot be maintained without an abundance of oxygen in the air we breathe.

This is of vital importance at all times, but especially so in acute disease, because here, as we have learned, all the vital processes are intensified. The system is working under high pressure. Large quantities of waste and morbid materials, the products of inflam-mation, have to be oxidized, that is, burned up and eliminated from the system.

In this respect the Nature Cure people have brought about one of the greatest reforms in medical treatment: the admission of plenty of fresh air to the sickroom.

But, strange to say, the importance of this most essential natural remedy is as yet not universally recognized by the representatives of the regular school of medicine. Time and again I have been called to sickrooms where by order of the doctor every window was closed and the room filled with pestilential odors, the poisonous exhalations of the diseased organism added to the stale air of the unventilated and often overheated apartment. And this air starvation had been enforced by graduates of our best medical schools and colleges. This unnatural and inexcusable crime against the sick is committed even at this late day in our great hospitals under the direct supervision of physicians who are foremost in their profession.

It is not the cold draft that is to be feared in the sickroom. Cool air is most agreeable and beneficial to the body burning in fever heat. What is to be feared is the reinhalation and reabsorption of poisonous emanations from the lungs and skin of the diseased body.

Furthermore, the ventilation of a room can be so regulated as to provide a constant and plentiful supply of fresh air without expos-ing its occupants to a direct draft. Where there is only one window and one door, both may be opened and a sheet or blanket hung across the opening of the door, or the single window may be opened partly from above and partly from below, which insures the entrance of fresh, cold air at the bottom and the expulsion of the heated and vitiated air at the top. The patient may be protected by a screen, or a board may be placed across the lower part of the window in such manner that a direct current of air upon the patient is prevented.

In very cold weather, or if conditions are not favorable to constant ventilation of the sickroom, the doors and windows may be opened wide for several minutes every few hours, while the patient's body and head are well protected. There is absolutely no danger of taking cold if these precautions are taken. Under right conditions of room temperature, frequent exposure of the patient's nude body to air and the sunlight will be found most beneficial and will often induce sleep when other means fail.

I would strongly warn against keeping the patient too warm. This is especially dangerous in the case of young children, who cannot use their own judgment or make their wishes known. I have frequently found children in high fever smothered in heavy blankets under the mistaken impression on the part of the attendants that they had to be kept warm and protected against possible draft. In many instances the air under the covers was actually steaming hot. This surely does not tend to reduce the burning fever heat in the body of the patient.

"Natural Diet" in Acute Diseases

From the appearance of the first suspicious symptoms until the fever has abated and there is a hearty, natural hunger, feeding should be reduced to a minimum or better still, entirely suspended.

In cases of extreme weakness, and where the acute and subacute processes are long drawn out and the patient has become greatly emaciated, it is advisable to give such easily digestible foods as white of egg, milk, buttermilk and whole grain bread with butter in combination with raw and stewed fruits and with vegetable salads prepared with lemon juice and olive oil.

The quantity of drinking water should be regulated by the desire of the patient, but he should be warned not to take any more than is necessary to satisfy his thirst. Large amounts of water taken into the system dilute the blood and the other fluids and secretions of the organism to an excessive degree, and this tends to increase the general weakness and lower the patient's resistance to the disease forces.

Water may be made more palatable and at the same time more effective for purposes of elimination by the addition of the unsweetened juice of acid fruits, such as orange, grapefruit or lemon, about one part of juice to three parts of water. Fresh pineapple juice is very good except in cases of hyperacidity of the stomach. The fresh, unsweetened juice of Concord grapes is also beneficial.

Acid and subacid fruit juices do not contain sufficient carbohydrate or protein materials to unduly excite the digestive processes, while on the other hand they are very rich in Nature's best medicines, the mineral salts in organic form. Sweet grapes and sweetened grape juice should not be given to patients suffering from acute, febrile diseases because they contain too much sugar, which would have a tendency to start the processes of digestion and assimilation, to cause morbid fermentation and to raise the temperature and accelerate the other disease symptoms.

Fasting

Total abstinence from food during acute febrile conditions is of primary importance. In certain diseases which will be mentioned later on, especially those involving the digestive tract, fasting must be continued for several days after all fever symptoms have disappeared.

There is no greater fallacy than that the patient must be sustained and his strength kept up by plenty of nourishing food and drink or, worse still, by stimulants and tonics. This is altogether wrong in itself, and besides, habit and appetite are often mistaken for hunger.

A common spectacle witnessed at the bedside of the sick is that of well-meaning but misguided relatives and friends forcing food and drink on the patient, often by order of the doctor, when his whole system rebels against it and the nauseated stomach expels the food as soon as taken. Sedatives and tonics are then resorted to in order to force the digestive organs into submission.

Aversion to eating during acute diseases, whether they represent healing crises or disease crises, is perfectly natural, because the entire organism, including the mucous membranes of stomach and intestines, is engaged in the work of elimination, not assimilation. Nausea, slimy and fetid discharges, constipation alternating with diarrhea, etc., indicate that the organs of digestion are throwing off disease matter, and that they are not in a condition to take up and assimilate food.

Ordinarily, the digestive tract acts like a sponge which absorbs the elements of nutrition; but in acute diseases the process is reversed, the sponge is being squeezed and gives off large quantities of morbid matter. The processes of digestion and assimilation are at a standstill. In fact, the entire organism is in a condition of prostration, weakness and inactivity. The vital energies are concentrated on the cleansing and healing processes. Accordingly, there is no demand for food.

This is verified by the fact that a person fasting for a certain period, say, four weeks, during the course of a serious acute illness, will not lose nearly as much in weight as the same person fasting four weeks in days of healthful activity.

It is for the foregoing reasons that nourishment taken during acute disease is not properly digested, assimilated and transmuted into healthy blood and tissues. Instead, it ferments and decays, filling the system with waste matter and noxious gases. interferes seriously with the elimination of morbid matter through stomach and intestines by forcing these organs to take up the work of digestion and assimilation. diverts the vital forces from their combat against the disease conditions and draws upon them to remove the worse than useless food ballast from the organism.

This explains why taking food during feverish diseases is usually followed by a rise in temperature and by aggravation of the other disease symptoms. As long as there are signs of inflammatory, febrile conditions and no appetite, do not be afraid to withhold food entirely, if necessary, for as long as five, six or seven weeks. In my practice I have had several patients who did not take any food, except water to which acid fruit juices had been added, for more than seven weeks, and then made a rapid and complete recovery.

In cases of gastritis, appendicitis, peritonitis, dysentery or typhoid fever, abstinence from food is absolutely imperative. Not even milk should be taken until fever and inflammation have entirely subsided, and then a few days should be allowed for the healing and restoring of the injured tissues. Many of the serious chronic aftereffects of these diseases are due to too early feeding, which does not allow the healing forces of Nature time to rebuild sloughed membranes and injured organs.

After a prolonged fast, great care must be observed when commencing to eat. Very small quantities of light food may safely be taken at intervals of a few hours. A good plan, especially after an attack of typhoid fever or dysentery, is to break the fast by thoroughly masticating one or two tablespoonfuls of popcorn. This gives the digestive tract a good scouring and starts the peristaltic action of the bowels better than any other food.

The popcorn may advantageously be followed in about two hours with a tablespoonful of cooked rice and one or two cooked prunes or a small quantity of some other stewed fruit.

For several days or weeks after a fast, according to the severity of the acute disease or healing crisis, a diet consisting largely of raw fruits, such as oranges, grapefruit, apples, pears, grapes, etc., and juicy vegetables, especially lettuce, celery, cabbage slaw, watercress, young onions, tomatoes or cucumbers should be adhered to. No condiments or dressings should be used with the vegetables except lemon juice and olive oil.

Hydropathic Treatment in Acute Diseases

We claim that in acute diseases hydropathic treatment will accomplish all the benefcial effects which the "Old School" practitioners ascribe to drugs, and that water applications will produce the desired results much more efficiently, and without any harmful by-effects or aftereffects upon the system.

The principal objects to be attained in the treatment of acute inflammatory diseases are:

To relieve the inner congestion and consequent pain in the affected parts. To keep the temperature below the danger point by promoting heat radiation through the skin. To increase the activity of the organs of elimination and thus to facilitate the removal of morbid materials from the system. To increase the positive electromagnetic energies in the organism. To increase the amount of oxygen and ozone in the system and thereby to promote the oxidation and combustion of effete matter.

The above-mentioned objects can be attained most effectually by the simple cold water treatment. Whatever the acute condition may be, whether an ordinary cold or the most serious type of febrile disease, the applications described in detail in the following pages, used singly, combined or alternately according to individual conditions, will always be in order and sufficient to produce the best possible results.

Baths and Ablutions

Cooling sprays or, if the patient is too weak to leave the bed, cold sponge baths or ablutions, repeated whenever the temperature rises, are very effective for keeping the fever below the danger point, for relieving the congestion in the interior of the body and for stimulating the elimination of systemic poisons through the skin.

However, care must be taken not to lower the temperature too much by the excessive coldness or unduly prolonged duration of the application. It is possible to suppress inflammatory processes by means of cold water or ice bags just as easily as with poisonous antiseptics, antifever medicines and surgical operations.

It is sufficient to reduce the temperature to just below the danger point. This will allow the inflammatory processes to run their natural course through the five progressive stages of inflammation and this natural course will then be followed by perfect regeneration of the affected parts.

In our sanitarium we use only water of ordinary temperature as it flows from the faucet, never under any circumstances ice bags or ice water. The application of ice keeps the parts to which it is applied in a chilled condition. The circulation cannot react, and the inflammatory processes are thus most effectually suppressed.

To recapitulate: Never check or suppress a fever by means of cold baths, ablutions, wet packs, etc., but merely lower it below the danger point. For instance, if a certain type of fever has a tendency to rise to 104 degree F. or more, bring it down to about 102 degree. If the fever ordinarily runs at a lower temperature, say at 102 degree F., do not try to reduce it more than one or two degrees.

If the temperature is subnormal, that is, below the normal or regular body temperature, the packs should be applied in such a manner that a warming effect is produced, that is, less wet cloths and more dry covering should be used, and the packs left on the body a longer time before they are renewed. More detailed instruction will be given in subsequent pages.

Never lose sight of the fact that fever is in itself a healing, cleansing process which must not be checked or suppressed.

Hot-Water Applications Are Injurious

Altogether wrong is the application of hot water to seats of inflammation as, for instance, the inflamed appendix or ovaries, sprains, bruises, etc. Almost in every instance where I am called in to attend a case of acute appendicitis or peritonitis, I find hot compresses or hot water bottles, by means of which the inflamed parts are kept continually in an overheated condition. It is in this way that a simple inflammation is nurtured into an abscess and made more serious and dangerous.

The hot compress or hot-water bottle draws the blood away from the inflamed area to the surface temporarily; but unless the hot application is kept up continually, the blood, under the Law of Action and Reaction, will recede from the surface into the interior, and as a result the inner congestion will become as great as or greater than before.

If the hot applications are continued, the applied heat tends to maintain and increase the heat in the inflamed parts.

Inflammation means that there is already too much heat in the affected part or organ. Common sense, therefore, would dictate cooling applications instead of heating ones.

The cold packs and compresses, on the other hand, have a directly cooling effect upon the seat of inflammation and in accordance with the Law of Action and Reaction their secondary, lasting effect consists in drawing the blood from the congested and heated interior to the surface, thus relaxing the pores of the skin and promoting the radiation of heat and the elimination of impurities.

Both the hot-water applications and the use of ice are, therefore, to be absolutely condemned. The only rational and natural treatment of inflammatory conditions is that by compresses, packs and ablutions, using water of ordinary temperature, as it comes from the cold water tap.

By means of the simple cold-water treatment and fasting all fevers and inflammations can be reduced in a perfectly natural way within a short time without undue strain on the organism.

The Whole-Body Pack

The whole-body pack is most effective if by means of it the patient can be brought into a state of copious perspiration. The pack is then removed and the patient is given a cold sponge bath.

It will be found that this treatment often produces a second profuse sweat which is very beneficial. This aftersweat should also be followed by a cold sponge bath.

Such a course of treatment will frequently be sufficient to eliminate the morbid matter which has gathered in the system, and thus prevent in a perfectly natural manner a threatening disease which otherwise might become dangerous to life.

How to Apply the Whole-Body Pack

On a bed or cot spread two or more blankets, according to their weight. Over the top blanket spread a linen or cotton sheet which has been dipped into cold water and wrung out fairly dry. Let the blankets extend about one foot beyond the wet sheet at the head of the bed.

Place the patient on the wet sheet so that it comes well up to the neck, and wrap the sheet snugly around the body so that it covers every part, tucking it in between the arms and sides and between the legs. It will be found that the sheet can be adjusted more snugly and smoothly if separate strips of wet linen are placed between the legs and between the arms and the sides of the body.

The blankets are now folded, one by one, upward over the feet and around the body, turned in at the neck and brought across the chest, the outer layers being held in place with safety pins.

The patient should stay in this whole-body pack from one-half hour to two hours, according to the object to be attained and the reaction of the body to the pack. If the pack has been correctly applied, the patient will become warm in a few minutes.

The Bed-Sweat Bath

If the patient does not react to the pack, that is, if he remains cold, or if, as is sometimes the case in malaria, the fever is accompanied by chills or if profuse perspiration is desired, bottles filled with hot water or bricks heated in the oven and wrapped in flannel should be placed along the sides and to the feet, under the outside covering.

This form of application is called the bed-sweat bath. It may be used with good results when an incipient cold is to be aborted.

After the pack has been removed, the body should be sponged with cold water, as already stated. Use a coarse cloth or Turkish towel for this purpose rather than a sponge, as the latter cannot be kept perfectly clean. Dry the body quickly but thoroughly, and finish by rubbing with the hands.

In the meantime the damp bed clothing should be replaced by dry sheets and blankets (a second cot or bed will be found a great convenience), and the patient put to bed without delay and well covered in order to prevent chilling and also to induce, if possible, a copious aftersweat. The patient is then sponged off a second time, put into a dry bed, and allowed to rest.

If the patient is too weak to leave his bed, the cold sponge may be given on a large rubber sheet or oilcloth covered with an old blanket, which should be placed on the bed before the pack is applied. After removing the pack, put a blanket over the patient to prevent chilling and wash quickly but thoroughly first the limbs, then chest and stomach, then the back, drying and covering each part as soon as finished. Remove the rubber sheet from the bed and wrap the patient in dry, warm blankets, or lift him into another bed.

How to Apply the Short-Body Pack

A wide strip of linen or muslin, wrung out of cold water, is wrapped around the patient from under the armpits to the thighs or knees in one, two or more layers, covered by one or more layers of dry flannel or muslin in such a manner that the wet linen does not protrude at any place.

Similar packs may be applied to the throat,* the arms, legs, shoulder joints or any other part of the body.

The number of layers of wet linen and dry covering is determined by the vitality of the patient, the height of his temperature and the particular object of the application, which may be to lower high temperature to raise the temperature when subnormal to relieve inner congestion to promote elimination.

If the object is to lower high temperature, several layers of wet linen should be wrapped around the body and covered loosely by one or two layers of the dry wrappings in order to prevent the bed from getting wet. The packs must be renewed as soon as they become dry or uncomfortably hot.

If the object is to raise subnormal temperature, less wet linen and more dry covering must be used, and the packs left on a longer time, say from thirty minutes to two hours. If the patient does not react to the pack, hot bricks or bottles filled with hot water should be placed at the sides and to the feet, as explained in connection with the whole-body pack.

If inner congestion is to be relieved, or if the object is to promote elimination, less of the wet linen and more dry wrappings should be used.

When packs are applied, the bed may be protected by spreading an oilcloth over the mattress under the sheet. But in no case should oilcloth or rubber sheeting be used for the outer covering of packs. This would interfere with some of the main objects of the pack treatment, especially with heat radiation. The outer covering should be warm but at the same time porous, to allow the escape of heat and of poisonous gases from the body.

Local Compresses

In case of local inflammation, as in appendicitis, ovaritis, colitis, etc., separate cooling compresses may be slipped under the pack and over the seat of inflammation. These local compresses may be removed and changed when hot and dry without disturbing the larger pack.

In all fevers accompanied by high temperature, it is advisable to place an extra cooling compress at the nape of the neck (the region of the medulla and the back brain), because here are located the brain centers which regulate the inner temperature of the body (thermotaxic centers), and the cooling of these brain centers produces a cooling effect upon the entire organism.

Enemas

While ordinarily we do not favor the giving of injections or enemas unless they are absolutely necessary, we apply them freely in feverish diseases in order to remove from the rectum and lower colon any accumulations of morbid matter, and thus to prevent their reabsorption into the system. In cases of exceptionally stubborn constipation, an injection of a few ounces of warm olive oil may be given. Allow this to remain in the colon about thirty minutes in order to soften the contents of the rectum, and follow with an injection of warm water.

Just How the Cold Packs Produce

Their Wonderful Results

(1) How Cold Packs Promote Heat Radiation

Many people are under the impression that the packs reduce the fever temperature so quickly because they are put on cold. But this is not so, because, unless the reaction be bad, the packs become warm after a few minutes' contact with the body.

The prompt reduction of temperature takes place because of increased heat radiation. The coldness of the pack may lower the surface temperature slightly; but it is the moist warmth forming under the pack on the surface of the body that draws the blood from the congested interior into the skin, relaxes and opens its minute blood vessels and pores, and in that way facilitates the escape of heat from the body.

In febrile conditions the pores and capillary blood vessels of the skin are tense and contracted. Therefore the heat cannot escape, the skin is hot and dry, and the interior of the body remains overheated. When the skin relaxes and the patient begins to perspire freely, we say the fever is broken.

The moist warmth under the wet pack produces this relaxation of the skin in a perfectly natural manner. By means of these simple packs followed by cold ablutions, the temperature of the patient can be kept at any point desired without the use of poisonous antifever medicines, serums and antitoxins which lower the temperature by benumbing and paralyzing heart action, respiration, the red and white blood corpuscles, and thus generally lowering the vital activities of the organism.

(2) How Cold Packs Relieve Inner Congestion

In all inflammatory febrile diseases the blood is congested in the inflamed parts and organs. This produces the four cardinal symptoms of inflammation: redness, swelling, heat, and pain. [Rubor, tumor, colar and dolar.] If the congestion be too great, the pain becomes excessive, and the inflammatory processes cannot run their natural course to the best advantage. It is therefore of great importance to relieve the local blood pressure in the affected parts and this can be accomplished most effectively by means of the wet packs.

As before stated, they draw the blood onto the surface of the body and in that way relieve inner congestion wherever it may exist, whether it be in the brain, as in meningitis, in the lungs, as in pneumonia, or in the inflamed appendix.

In several cases where a child was in the most dangerous stage of diphtheria, where the membranes in throat and nasal passages were already choking the little patient, the wet packs applied to the entire body from neck to feet relieved the congestion in the throat so quickly that within half an hour after the first application the patient breathed easily and soon made a perfect recovery. The effectiveness of these simple water applications in reducing congestion, heat and pain is little short of marvelous.

(3) How Cold Packs Promote Elimination

By far the largest number of deaths in febrile diseases result from the accumulation in the system of poisonous substances, which paralyze or destroy vital centers and organs. Therefore it is necessary to eliminate the morbid products of inflammation from the organism as quickly as possible.

This also is accomplished most effectively and thoroughly by the application of wet packs. As they draw the blood into the surface and relax the minute blood vessels in the skin, the morbid materials in the blood are eliminated through the pores of the skin and absorbed by the packs. That this is actually so is verified by the yellowish or brownish discoloration of the wet wrappings and by their offensive odor.

One of the main causes of constipation in febrile diseases is the inner congestion and fever heat. Through the cooling and relaxing effect of the packs upon the intestines, this inner fever heat is reduced, and a natural movement of the bowels greatly facilitated.

If constipation should persist in spite of the packs and cooling compresses, injections of tepid water should be given every day or every other day in order to prevent the reabsorption of poisonous products from the lower colon. But never give injections of cold water with the idea of reducing fever in that way. This is very dangerous and may cause fatal collapse.

The Electromagnetic Effect of

Cold Water Applications

One of the most important, but least understood, effects of hydropathic treatment is its influence upon the electromagnetic energies in the human body. At least, I have never found any allusions to this aspect of the cold-water treatment in any books on hydrotherapy which have come to my notice.

The sudden application of cold water or cold air to the surface of the nude body and the inhalation of cold air into the lungs have the effect of increasing the amount of electromagnetic energy in the system.

This can be verified by the following experiment: Insert one of the plates of an electrometer (sensitive galvanometer) into the stomach of a person who has remained for some time in a warm room. Now let this person inhale suddenly fresh, cold outside air. At once the galvanometer will register a larger amount of electromagnetic energy.

The same effect will be produced by the application of a quick, cold spray to the warm body.

It is the sudden lowering of temperature on the surface of the body or in the lungs and the resulting contrast between the heat within and the cold outside, that causes the increased manifestation of electromagnetic energy in the system.

This, together with the acceleration of the entire circulation, undoubtedly accounts for the tonic effect of cold-water applications such as cold packs, ablutions, sprays, sitz baths, barefoot walking, etc., and for the wonderfully bracing influence of fresh, cold outside air.

The energizing effect of cold air may also explain to a large extent the superiority of the races inhabiting the temperate zones over those of the warm and torrid southern regions.

To me it seems a very foolish custom to run away from the invigorating northern winters to the enervating sameness of southern climates. One of the reasons I abandoned, with considerable financial sacrifice, a well-established home in a Texas city which is the Mecca of health-seekers, was that I did not want to rear my children under the enervating influence of that beautiful climate. I, for my part, want some cold winter weather every year to stir up the lazy blood corpuscles, to set the blood bounding through the system and to freeze out the microbes.

In our Nature Cure work we find all the way through that the continued application of warmth has a debilitating effect upon the organism, and that only by the opposing influences of alternating heat and cold can we produce the natural stimulation which awakens the dormant vital energies in the body of the chronic.

Increase of Oxygen and Ozone

The liberation of electromagnetic currents through cold-water applications has other very important effects upon the system besides that of stimulation.

Electricity splits up molecules of water into hydrogen, oxygen and ozone. We have an example of this in the thunderstorm. The powerful electric discharges which we call lightning separate or split the watery vapors in the air into these elements. It is the increase of oxygen and ozone in the air that purifies and sweetens the atmosphere after the storm.

In acute as well as in chronic disease, large amounts of oxygen and ozone are required to burn up the morbid materials and to purify the system. Certain combinations of these elements are among the most powerful antiseptics and germicides.

Likewise, the electric currents produced by cold packs, ablutions and other cold-water applications split up the molecules of water in the tissues of the body into their component parts. In this way large amounts of oxygen and ozone are liberated, and these elements assist to a considerable extent in the oxidation and neutralization of waste materials and disease products.

The following experiment proves that sudden changes in temperature create electric currents in metals: When two cylinders of dissimilar metals are welded together, and one of the metals is suddenly chilled or heated, electric currents are produced which will continue to flow until both metals are at the same temperature.

Another application of this principle is furnished by the oxydonor. If both poles of this little instrument are exposed to the same temperature, there is no manifestation of electricity; but if one of the poles be attached to the warm body and the other immersed in cold water or exposed to cold air, the liberation of electromagnetic currents begins at once. These electric currents set free oxygen and ozone, which in their turn support the oxidation and neutralization of systemic poisons.

According to my experience, however, the cold-water applications are more effective in this respect than the oxydonor.

The Importance of Right Mental and Emotional Attitude in Acute Disease

We have learned that in the processes of inflammation a battle is going on between the healing forces of the body, the phagocytes and natural antitoxins on the one hand and the disease taints, germs, bacilli, etc., on the other hand.

This battle is real in every respect, as real as a combat between armies of living soldiers. In this conflict, going on in all acute inflammatory diseases, mind plays the same role as the commander of an army.

The great general needs courage, equanimity and presence of mind most in the stress of battle. So the mind, the commander of the vast armies of cells battling in acute disease for the health of the body, must have absolute faith in the superiority of Nature's healing forces.

If the mind becomes frightened by the inflammatory and febrile symptoms and pictures to itself in darkest colors their dreadful consequences, these confused and distracted thought vibrations are conveyed instantaneously to the millions of little soldiers fighting in the affected parts and organs. They also become confused and panic-stricken.

The excitement of fear in the mind still more accelerates heart action and respiration, intensifies the local congestion and greatly increases the morbid accumulations in the system. In the last chapters of this volume we shall deal especially with the deteriorating influence of fear, anxiety, anger, irritability, impatience, etc., and explain how these and all other destructive emotions actually poison the secretions of the body.

In acute disease we cannot afford to add to the poisonous elements in the organism, because the danger of a fatal ending lies largely in the paralysis of vital centers by the morbid and poisonous products of inflammation.

Everything depends upon the maintenance of the greatest possible inflow of vital force; and there is nothing so weakening as worry and anxiety, nothing that impedes the inflow, distribution and normal activity of the vital energies like fear. A person overcome by sudden fright is actually benumbed and paralyzed, unable to think and to act intelligently.

These truths may be expressed in another way. The victory of the healing forces in acute disease depends upon an abundant supply of the positive electromagnetie energies. In the initial chapters of this volume we have learned that health is positive, disease negative. The positive mental attitude of faith and equanimity creates positive electromagnetic energies in the body, thus infusing the battling phagocytes with increased vigor and favoring the secretion of the antitoxins and antibodies, while the negative, fearful and worrying attitude of mind creates in the system the negative conditions of weakness, lowered resistance and actual paralysis.

In the paragraphs dealing with the effects of cold-water treatment upon the body we learned that the electric currents created in the organism split up the molecules of water in the tissues into their component elements (hydrogen and oxygen), thus liberating large amounts of oxygen and ozone; and that these, in turn, support the processes of combustion and oxidation in the system, burn up waste and morbid matter, and destroy hostile microorganisms.

However, the electromagnetic forces in the body are not only increased and intensified by positive foods, exercise, cold-water treatment, air baths, etc., but also by the positive attitude of mind and will.

The positive mind and will are to the body what the magneto is to the automobile. As the electric sparks from the magneto ignite the gas, thus generating the power that drives the machine, so the positive vibrations, generated by a confident and determined will, create in the body the positive electromagnetic currents which incite and stimulate all vital activities.

Common experience teaches us that the concentration of the will on the thing to be accomplished greatly heightens and increases all physical, mental and moral powers.

Therefore the victory in acute diseases is conditioned by the absolute faith, confidence and serenity of mind on the part of the patient. The more he exercises these harmonizing and invigorating qualities of mind and soul, the more favorable are the conditions for the little soldiers who are fighting his battles in the inflamed parts and organs. The blood and nerve currents are less impeded and disturbed, and flow more normally. The local congestion is relieved, and this favors the natural course of the inflammatory processes.

Therefore, instead of being overcome with fear and anxiety, as most people are under such circumstances, do not become alarmed, nor convey alarm to the millions of little cells battling in the inflamed parts. Speak to them like a commander addressing his troops: "We understand the laws of disease and cure, we know that these inflammatory and febrile symptoms are the result of Nature's healing efforts, we have perfect confidence in her wisdom and in the efficiency of her healing forces. This fever is merely a good house-cleaning, a healing crisis. We are eliminating morbid matter, poisons and germs which were endangering health and life.

"We rejoice over the purification and regeneration now taking place and benefiting the whole body. Fear not! Attend to your work quietly and serenely! Let us open ourselves wide to the inflow of life from the source of all life in the innermost parts of our being! The life in us is the life of God. We are strengthened and made whole by the Divine life and power which animate the universe."

The serenity of your mind, backed by absolute trust in the Law and by the power of a strong Will, infuses the cells and tissues with new life and vigor, enabling them to turn the acute disease into a beneficial, cleansing and healing crisis.

In the following we give a similar formula for treating chronic constipation.

Say to the cells in the liver, the pancreas and the intestinal tract:

"I am not going to force you any longer with drugs or enemas to do your duty. From now on you must work on your own initiative. Your secretions will become more abundant. Every day at—o'clock the bowels will move freely and easily."

At the appointed time make the effort, whether you are success-ful or not, and do not resort to the enema until it becomes an absolute necessity. If you combine with the mental and physical effort a natural diet, cold sitz baths, massage and osteopathic treatment, you will have need of the enema at increasingly longer intervals, and soon be able to discard it altogether.

Be careful, however, not to employ your intelligence and your will power to suppress acute inflammatory and febrile processes and symptoms. This can be accomplished by the power of the will as well as by ice bags and poisonous drugs, and its effect would be to turn Nature's acute cleansing efforts into chronic disease.

The Importance of Right Mental and Emotional

Attitude on the Part of Friends and Relatives

What has just been said about the patient is true also of his friends and relatives. Disease is negative. The sick person is exceedingly sensitive to his surroundings. He is easily influenced by all depressing, discordant and jarring conditions. He catches the expressions of fear and anxiety in the looks, the words, gestures and actions of his attendants, relatives and friends and these intensify his own depression and gloomy forebodings.

This applies especially to the influence exerted by the mother upon her ailing infant. There exists a most intimate sympathetic and telepathic connection between mother and child. The child is affected not only by the outward expression of the mother's fear and anxiety, but likewise by the hidden doubt and despair in the mother's mind and soul.

Usually, the first thing that confronts me when I am called to the sickbed of a child is the frantic and almost hysterical mental condition of the mother, and to begin with, I have to explain to her the destructive influence of her behavior. I ask her:

"Would you willingly give some deadly poison to your child?"
"Certainly not," she says, to which I reply:

"Do you realize that you are doing this very thing? That your fear and worry vibrations actually poison and paralyze the vital energies in the body of your child and most seriously interfere with Nature's healing processes?

"Instead of helping the disease forces to destroy your child, assist the healing forces to save it by maintaining an attitude of absolute faith, serenity, calmness and cheerfulness. Then your looks, your voice, your touch will convey to your child the positive, magnetic vibrations of health and of strength. Your very presence will radiate healing power."

Then I explain how faith, calmness and cheerfulness on her part will soothe and harmonize the discordant disease vibrations in the child's body.

Herein lies the modus operandi or working basis of all successful mental and metaphysical treatment.

Summary

Natural Methods in the Treatment of Acute Disease

~I. Fresh Air~

A plentiful supply of pure air in the sickroom. Frequent exposure of the nude body to air and sun light. Patient must not be kept too warm.

~II. Natural Diet~

The minimum amount of light food, chiefly fruit and vegetable salads, no condiments. Only enough water to quench thirst, preferably mixed with acid fruit juices. In serious acute febrile conditions and during healing crises no food whatever. In diseases affecting the digestive organs fasting must be prolonged several days beyond cessation of febrile symptoms. Great care must be observed when breaking fast.

~III. Water Treatment~

Cooling sprays or sponge baths whenever temperature rises. Fever and inflammation must not be suppressed by cold-water applications, but kept below the danger point. Neither ice nor hot applications should be used. Wet packs followed by cold ablutions for elimination of systemic poisons. Separate compresses over seat of inflammation, also at nape of neck. Kind and duration of pack to be determined by condition of patient and object to be attained. Injections of tepid water to relieve constipation when necessary.

~IV. Medications~

No poisonous drugs, nor any medicines or applications which may check or suppress the feverish, inflammatory processes. Homeopathic medicines, herb decoctions and specific nutritional remedies when indicated.

~V. Manipulative Treatment~

Osteopathy, massage or magnetic treatment when indicated and available.

~VI. Mental Attitude~

Courage, serenity and presence of mind are important factors. Fear and anxiety intensify disease conditions, poison the secretions of the body and inhibit the action of the healing forces. Do not suppress acute inflammatory and feverish processes by the power of the will. The right mental and emotional attitude of relatives and friends exerts a powerful influence upon the patient.

Chapter XIV

The True Scope of Medicine

Anyone able to read the signs of the times cannot help observing the powerful influence which the Nature Cure philosophy is already exerting upon the trend of modern medical science. In Germany the younger generation of physicians has been forced by public demand to adopt the natural methods of treatment and the German government has introduced them in the medical departments of its army and navy.

In English-speaking countries, the foremost members of the medical profession are beginning to talk straight Nature Cure doctrine, to condemn the use of drugs and to endorse unqualifiedly the Nature Cure methods of treatment. In proof of this I quote from an article by Dr. William Osler in the ~Encyclopedia Americana,~ Vol. X, under the title of "Medicine":

Dr. Osler on Medicine

"The new school does not feel itself under obligation to give any medicines whatever, while a generation ago not only could few physicians have held their practice unless they did, but few would have thought it safe or scientific. Of course, there are still many cases where the patient or the patient's friends must be humored by administering medicine or alleged medicine where it is not really needed, and indeed often where the buoyancy of mind which is the real curative agent, can only be created by making him wait hopefully for the expected action of medicine; and some physicians still cannot unlearn their old training. But the change is great. The modern treatment of disease relies very greatly on the old so-called natural methods, diet and exercise, bathing and massage—in other words, giving the natural forces the fullest scope by easy and thorough nutrition, increased flow of blood and removal of obstructions to the excretory systems or the circulation in the tissues.

"One notable example is typhoid fever. At the outset of the nineteenth century it was treated with 'remedies' of the extremest violence—bleeding and blistering, vomiting and purging, and the administration of antimony and mercury, and plenty of other heroic remedies. Now the patient is bathed and nursed and carefully tended, but rarely given medicine. This is the result partly of the remarkable experiments of the Paris and Vienna schools in the action of drugs, which have shaken the stoutest faiths; and partly of the constant and reproachful object lesson of homeopathy. No regular physician would ever admit that the homeopathic preparations, 'infinitesimals,' could do any good as direct curative agents; and yet it was perfectly certain that homeopaths lost no more of their patients than others. There was but one conclusion to draw—that most drugs had no effect whatever on the diseases for which they were administered."

Dr. Osler is probably the greatest medical authority on drugs now living. He was formerly professor of materia medica at the Johns Hopkins University of Baltimore, U. S., and now holds a professorship at Oxford University, England. His books on medical practice are in use in probably every university and medical school in English-speaking countries. His views on drugs and their real value as expressed in this article should be an eye-opener to those good people who believe that we of the Nature Cure school are altogether too radical, extreme, and somewhat cranky.

However, what Dr. Osler says regarding the "New School" is true only of a few advanced members of the medical profession.

On the rank and file, the idea of drugless healing has about the same effect as a red rag on a mad bull. There are still very few physicians in general practice today who would not lose their bread and butter if they attempted to practice drugless healing on their patients. Both the profession and the public will need a good deal more education along Nature Cure lines before they will see the light.

In the second sentence of his article, Dr. Osler admits the efficacy of mental therapeutics and therapeutic faith as a "curative agent," and ascribes the good effects of medicine to their stimulating influence upon the patient's mind rather than to any beneficial action of the drugs themselves.

With regard to the origin of the modern treatment of typhoid fever, however, the learned doctor is either misinformed or he misrepresents the facts. The credit for the introduction of hydropathic treatment of typhoid fever does not belong to the "remarkable experiments of the Paris and Vienna schools." These schools and the entire medical profession fought this treatment with might and main. For thirty years Priessnitz, Bilz, Ruhne, Father Kneipp and many other pioneers of Nature Cure were persecuted and prosecuted, dragged into the courts and tried on the charges of malpractice and manslaughter for using their sane and natural methods. Not until Dr. Braun of Berlin wrote an essay on the good results obtained by the hydropathic treatment of typhoid fever and it had in that way received orthodox baptism and sanction, was it adopted by advanced physicians all over the world.

Through the Nature Cure treatment of typhoid fever, the mortality of this disease has been reduced from over fifty percent under the old drug treatment to less than five percent under the water treatment.

But the average medical practitioner has not yet learned from the Nature Cure school, that the same simple fasting and cold water which cure typhoid fever so effectively, will just as surely and easily cure every other form of acute disease, as, for instance, scarlet fever, diphtheria, smallpox, cerebrospinal meningitis, appendicitis, etc. Therefore, we claim that there is no necessity for the employment of poisonous drugs, serums and antitoxins for this purpose.

Referring to the last two sentences of Dr. Osler's article, homeopaths have, as a matter of fact, lost less patients than allopaths. The effect of homeopathic medicine, moreover, is not altogether negative, as Dr. Osler implies. The discovery of the minute cell as the basis of the human organism on the one hand and of the unlimited divisibility of matter on the other hand explains the rationality of the infinitesimal dose. Health and disease are resident in the cell; therefore, the homeopath doctors the cell, and the size of the dose has to be apportioned to the size of the patient.

When Dr. Osler says that most drugs have no effect whatsoever, he makes a serious misstatement. While they may not contribute anything to the cure of the disease for which they are given, they are often very harmful in themselves.

Almost every virulent poison known to man is found in allopathic prescriptions. It is now positively proved by the Diagnosis from the Eye that these poisons have a tendency to accumulate in the system, to concentrate in certain parts and organs for which they have a special affinity and then to cause continual irritation and actual destruction of tissues. By far the greater part of all chronic diseases are created or complicated on the one hand by the suppression of acute diseases by means of drug poisons, and on the other hand through the destructive effects of the drugs themselves.

Dr. Schwenninger, the medical adviser of Prince Bismarck, and later of Richard Wagner, the great composer, has published a book entitled ~The Doctor.~ This work is the most scathing arraignment and condemnation of modern medical practice, especially of poisonous drugs and of surgery. Dr. Treves, the body physician of the late King Edward of England, is no less outspoken in his denunciation of drugging than Drs. Osler and Schwenninger.

Just a few men like these, foremost in the medical profession, who have achieved financial and scientific independence, can afford to speak so frankly. The great majority of physicians, even though they know better, continue in the old ruts so as to be considered ethical and orthodox, and in order to hold their practice. It is not the medical profession that has brought about this reform in the treatment of typhoid fever and other diseases. They have been forced into the adoption of the more advanced natural methods through the pressure of the Nature Cure movement in Germany and elsewhere.

Dr. Osler's statements, made with due deliberation in a contribution to the ~Encyclopedia Americana,~ are certainly a frank declaration as to the uselessness of drug treatment, and on the other hand, an unqualified endorsement of natural methods of healing.

But it seems to me that Dr. Osler pours out the baby with the bath water, as we say in German. That is, I am inclined to think that his opinion regarding the ineffectiveness of drugs is entirely too radical. There is a legitimate scope for medicinal remedies insofar as they build up the blood on a natural basis and serve as tissue foods.

Many people who have lost their faith in "Old School" methods of treatment have swung around to the other extreme of medical nihilism. In fact, Dr. Osler himself stands accused of being a medical nihilist.

Many of those who have adopted natural methods of living and of treating diseases have acquired an actual horror of the word medicine. However, this extreme attitude is not justified.

It also appears that some of the readers of my writings are under the impression that we of the Nature Cure school absolutely condemn the use of any and all medicines. This, however, is not so.

The Position of "Nature Cure" Regarding Medicinal Remedies

We do condemn the use of drugs insofar as they are poisonous and destructive and insofar as they suppress acute diseases or healing crises, which are Nature's cleansing and healing efforts; but on the other hand we realize that there is a wide field for the helpful application of medicinal remedies insofar as they act as foods to the tissues of the body and as neutralizers and eliminators of waste and morbid materials.

In every form of chronic disease there exists in the system, on the one hand, an excess of certain morbid materials, and on the other hand, a deficiency of certain mineral constituents, organic salts, which are essential to the normal functions of the body.

Thus, in all anemic diseases the blood is lacking in iron, which picks up the oxygen in the air cells of the lungs and carries it into the tissues, and in sodium, which combines with the carbonic acid (coalgas) that is constantly being liberated in the system and conveys it to the organs of depuration, especially the lungs and the skin. In point of fact, oxygen starvation is due in a much greater degree to the deficiency of sodium and the consequential accumulation of carbonic acid in the system (carbonic acid asphyxiation) than to the lack of iron in the blood, as assumed by the regular school of medicine.

Foods or medicinal remedies which will supply this deficiency of iron and sodium in the organism will tend to overcome the anemic conditions.

The great range of uric acid diseases, such as rheumatism, calculi, arteriosclerosis, certain forms of diabetes and albuminuria, are due, on the one hand, to the excessive use of acid-producing foods, and on the other hand, to a deficiency in the blood of certain alkaline mineral elements, especially sodium, magnesium and potassium, whose office it is to neutralize and eliminate the acids which are created and liberated in the processes of starchy and protein digestion.

In another chapter I have explained the origin and progressive development of uric-acid diseases. Our volume on Natural Dietetics will contain additional proof that practically all diseases are caused by, or complicated with, acid conditions in the system.

Any foods or medicines which will provide the system with sufficient quantities of the acid-binding, alkaline mineral salts will prove to be good medicine for all forms of acid diseases.

The mineral constituents necessary to the vital economy of the organism should, however, be supplied in the organic form. This will be explained more fully in subsequent pages.

From what I have said, it becomes apparent that it is impossible to draw a sharp line of distinction between foods and medicines. All foods which serve the above-named purposes are good medicines, and all nonpoisonous herb extracts, homeopathic and vitochemical remedies that have the same effect upon the system are, for the same reason, good foods.

The medical treatment of the Nature Cure school consists largely in the proper selection and combination of food materials. This must be so. It stands to reason that Nature has provided within the ranges of the natural foods all the elements which Man needs in the way of food and medicine.

But it is quite possible that, through continued abuse, the digestive apparatus has become so weak and so abnormal that it cannot function properly, that it cannot absorb and assimilate from natural foods a sufficient quantity of the elements which the organism needs. In such cases it may be very helpful and indeed imperative to take the organic mineral salts in the forms of fruit, herb and vegetable juices, extracts or decoctions. Among the best of these food remedies are extracts of leafy vegetables such as lettuce, spinach, Scotch kale, cabbage, Swiss chard, etc. These vegetables are richer than any other foods in the positive mineral salts. The extract may be prepared from one or more of these vegetables, according to the supply on hand or the tolerance of the digestive organs and the taste and preference of the patient. They should be ground to a pulp in a vegetable grinder, then pressed out in a small fruit press, which can be secured in any department store. One or two teacups per day will be sufficient to supply the needs of the system for mineral salts. This extract should be prepared fresh every day.

Then there are the Kneipp Herb Remedies. Most of these are the Hausmittel [home remedies] of the country population of Germany which have proved their efficacy since time immemorial. Their medicinal value lies in the organic mineral salts which they contain in large quantities and in beneficial combinations.

The homeopathic medications, as will be explained at length in another chapter, produce their good results because they work in harmony with the Laws of Nature.

We never hesitate, therefore, to prescribe for our patients homeopathic medicines, herb decoctions and extracts, and the vitochemical remedies which assist in the elimination of morbid matter from the system and in building up blood and lymph on a normal basis, that is, remedies which supply the organism with the mineral elements in which it is deficient in the organic, easily assimilable form. Herein lies the legitimate scope of medicinal remedies.

All medicinal remedies which build up the system on a normal, natural basis and increase its fighting power against disease without in any way inflicting injury upon the organism are welcome to the adherents of the Nature Cure methods of treatment.

On the other hand, we do not use any drugs or medicines which tend to hinder, check or suppress Nature's cleansing and regenerating processes. We never give anything in the least degree poisonous. We avoid all anodynes, hypnotics, sedatives, antipyretics, laxatives, cathartics, etc. Judicious fasting, cold-water applications and, if necessary, warm-water injections in case of constipation will do everything that is claimed for poisonous drugs.

Inorganic Minerals and Mineral Poisons

For many years past, physicians of the different schools of medicine, diet experts and food chemists have been divided on the question whether or not mineral substances which in the organic form enter into the composition of the human body may safely be used in foods and medicines in the inorganic form.

The medical profession holds almost unanimously that this is permissible and good practice, so that nearly every allopathic medical prescription contains some such inorganic substance, or worse than that, one or more virulent mineral poisons, as mercury, arsenic, phosphorus, etc.

So far, the discussion about the usefulness or harmfulness of inorganic minerals as foods and medicines was largely theoretical and controversial. Neither party had positive proofs for its contentions.

But Nature's records in the iris of the eye settle the question for good and for ever. One of the fundamental principles of the science of Diagnosis from the Eye is that "nothing shows in the iris by abnormal signs or discolorations except that which is abnormal in the body or injurious to it." When substances which are uncongenial or poisonous to the system accumulate in any part or organ of the body in sufficient quantities, they will indicate their presence by certain signs and abnormal colors in the corresponding areas of the iris.

In this way Nature makes known by her records in the eye what substances are injurious to the body, and which are harmless.

Certain mineral elements, such as iron, sodium, potassium, calcium, magnesium, phosphorus, sulphur, etc., which are among the important constituents of the human body, may be taken in the organic form in fruits and vegetables, or in herb extracts and the vitochemical remedies, in large amounts, in fact, far beyond the actual needs of the body, but they will not show in the iris of the eye, because they are easily eliminated from the system.

If, however, the same minerals be taken in the inorganic form in considerable quantities, the iris will exhibit certain well-defined signs and discolorations in the areas corresponding to those parts of the body in which the mineral substances have accumulated.

Obviously, Nature does not intend that these mineral elements should enter the organism in the inorganic form, and therefore the organs of depuration are not able to neutralize and eliminate them.

Thus, for instance, any amount of iron may be taken in vegetable or herb

This is proved by the fact that the signs of the minerals which are normal constituents of the human body disappear from the iris of the eye much more quickly than the signs of those minerals which are foreign and naturally poisonous to the system.

The difficulty we experience in eliminating mineral poisons from the body would seem to indicate that Nature never intended them to be used as foods or medicines. The intestines, kidneys, skin, mucous membranes and other organs of depuration are evidently not constructed or prepared to cope with inorganic, poisonous substances and to eliminate them completely. Accordingly, these poisons show the tendency to accumulate in certain parts or organs of the body for which they have a special affinity and then to act as irritants and destructive corrodents.

The diseases which we find most difficult to cure, even by the most radical application of natural methods, are cases of drug-poisoning. Substances which are foreign to the human organism, and especially the inorganic, mineral poisons, positively destroy tissues and organs, and are much harder to eliminate from the system than the encumbrances of morbid materials and waste matter produced in the body by wrong habits of living only. The obvious reason for this is that our organs of elimination are intended and constructed to excrete only such waste products as are formed in the organism in the processes of metabolism.

Tuberculosis or cancer may be caused in a scrofulous or psoriatic constitution by overloading the system with meat, coffee, alcohol or tobacco; but as soon as these bad habits are discontinued, and the organs of elimination stimulated by natural methods, the encumbrances will be eliminated, and the much-dreaded symptoms will subside and disappear, often with surprising rapidity.

On the other hand, mercury, arsenic, quinine, strychnine, iodine, etc., accumulate in the brain, the spinal cord, and the cells and tissues of the vital organs, causing actual destruction and disintegration. The tissues thus affected are not easily rebuilt, and it is exceedingly difficult to stir up the destructive mineral poisons and to eliminate them from the system.

Therefore it is an indisputable fact that many of the most stubborn, so-called incurable diseases are drug diseases

The Importance of Natural Diet

While certain medicinal remedies in organic form may be very useful in supplying quickly a deficiency of mineral elements in the system, we should aim to keep our bodies in a normal, healthy condition by proper food selection and combination. A brief description of the scientific basis of "Natural Dietetics" will be found in the chapter on Diet.

Undoubtedly, Nature has supplied all the elements which the human organism needs in abundance and in the right proportions in the natural foods, otherwise she would be a very ignorant organizer and provider.

We should learn to select and combine food materials in such a manner that they supply all the needs of the body in the best possible way and thus insure perfect health and strength without the use of medicines.

Why should we attempt to cure anemia with inorganic iron, hyperacidity of the stomach with baking soda, swollen glands with iodine, the itch with sulphur, ricket conditions in infants with lime water, etc., when these mineral elements are contained in abundance and in live, organic form in fruits and vegetables, herbs and in the vitochemical remedies?

Unfortunately, however, a great many individuals, through wrong habits of living and of treating their ailments, have ruined their digestive organs to such an extent that they are incapable of properly assimilating their food and require, at least temporarily, stimulative treatment by natural methods and a supply of the indispensable organic mineral salts through medicinal food preparations.

In such cases the mineral elements must be provided in the most easily assimilable form in vegetable extracts (which should be prepared fresh every day), and in the vitochemical remedies.

What has been said is sufficient, I believe, to justify the attitude of the Nature Cure school toward medicines in general. It explains why we avoid the use of inorganic minerals and poisonous substances, while on the other hand we find a wide and useful field for medicinal remedies in the form of blood and tissue foods.

www.ingramcontent.com/pod-product-compliance
Lightning Source LLC
Chambersburg PA
CBHW081722100526
44591CB00016B/2472